Dr. Paul Dougherty is the go-to eye surgeon for answers about the latest options in vision correction technology. His extensive professional experience, state-of-the-art training, and innovation of the latest lens and laser-based technologies, (plus having had vision correction surgery himself), place him in a unique position to help you sort out the many options now available for better vision without glasses or contacts.

Dr. Dougherty's technical and medical background, combined with his empathetic ability to communicate to people who want to improve their vision, shines through in this book. He writes with compassion, as if sitting across from a patient, expertly discussing the patient's individual vision concerns.

With crystal clarity, he describes how the eye works and the various vision conditions commonly faced, particularly as people age. He then explores the various options for vision improvement. He answers every question and dispels every concern about various vision correction techniques.

See for Yourself takes a close look at:

- How to select your eye surgeon
- The various techniques available—from LASIK to new lens-based vision correction alternatives including the new VISTA VISION ICL™ and beyond
- The future of vision correction
- Misconceptions surrounding vision correction

Dr. Dougherty's knowledge and understanding have earned him unique respect from both peers and patients. He is often called "the doctor's doctor" and is the surgeon frequently chosen by other physicians and eye care professionals for their own vision correction surgery. His book imparts hope to people who would like to see better. More importantly, it brings this hope based on a solid foundation of facts and experience.

SEE
FOR
YOURSELF

SEE
FOR
YOURSELF

THE EYE-OPENING
GUIDE TO PERMANENT
VISION CORRECTION

PAUL J. DOUGHERTY, MD

VISIONARY
PRESS

Los Angeles, CA

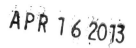

Visionary Press
321 N. Larchmont Blvd., Ste. 1021
Los Angeles, CA 90004
323.466.7338

Disclosure: The information presented in this book is not a substitute for professional medical advice. For medical advice about your eyes or vision, please contact your own eye care professional or make an appointment for a complimentary consultation with Dougherty Laser Vision at 866.987.2020 or www.doughertylaservision.com.

Printed in the United States of America, on acid-free paper.

Library of Congress Control Number: 2012932413

Publisher's Cataloguing-in-Publication Data
Dougherty, Paul J. (Paul Joseph), 1963-
See for yourself : the eye-opening guide to permanent vision correction / Paul J. Dougherty. -- Los Angeles, Calif. : Visionary Press, c2012.
p. ; cm.
ISBN: 978-0-9850390-0-4 (cloth) ; 978-0-9850390-1-1 (pbk.) ; 978-0-9850390-2-8 (ebk.)
Includes bibliographical references and index.
Summary: If you look at life through glasses or contact lenses, or if your vision is blurry, this book lays out options for vision correction so anyone can begin to make informed choices on what will serve them best.--Publisher.
1. Eye--Laser surgery--Popular works. 2. LASIK (Eye surgery)--Popular works. 3. Intraocular lenses--Popular works. I. Title.

RE86 .D68 2012   2012932413
617.7/1--dc23   1204

Book Consultant: Ellen Reid
Cover and Interior Design: Patricia Bacall
Author Photos: Starla Fortunato

Contents

Paul Dougherty is a visionary. He not only helps people see better, but sees how to serve many who cannot afford vision correction. He travels to foreign countries, teaching doctors the latest techniques of corrective surgery, and has operated on the eyes of countless underprivileged people, giving them both the gift of vision and the gift of his love.

In this book, Dr. Paul shows why LASIK is not for everyone and that there are alternative procedures that can allow all of us the best vision possible.

Some of my closest friends have trusted Dr. Paul with their eyes, and he has been both a friend and doctor to me. It is inspiring to see him give the same love and attention to those in need that he gives to his many celebrity clients.

Dr. Paul makes Happy Health. I love Dr. Paul. In Dr. Paul we trust.

Fred Segal

February 14, 2012
Santa Monica, California

Fred Segal is man of exceptional talent and faith, a pioneer of branding and fashion marketing, plus an honored peace and environmental activist and humanitarian.

For more information about this book:

www.seeforyourselfbook.com

Acknowledgments

Writing this book is the fulfillment of a lifelong dream that owes a tremendous debt to the time, energy, input, and patience of many people. I would first and foremost like to thank my friend and mentor, Craig Marshall Domigan, for his inspiration, expertise, and hard work that were so helpful in writing this book. Without him, this dream would never have become reality. I also credit Craig with helping me to understand that this life is but a dream — and what a wonderful dream it has been. I would also like to thank Rich Bains for his editing prowess with the manuscript after the initial drafts, as well as Randy Bissel for his friendship and support in efficiently running my businesses while I concentrated on finishing this book.

In addition, this book would not have been possible without the help of my world-class Book Shepherd/Producer, Ellen Reid, and her expert team who worked with Visionary Press, including Patricia Bacall, who designed the book, Starla Fortunato, who is responsible for the beautiful cover photos, Pamela Guerreri, who edited and proofread the manuscript, and Bruce Tracey, who indexed the book. Thanks also to Rona Menashe of Guttman and Associates for her friendship and advice on the manuscript and design. A heartfelt thank you also goes out to my dear daughter, Abigail, for her support in understanding the time commitment required in researching and writing this book as well as her hard work and creative expertise in designing the logo. In addition, I would like to thank my son Andrew for helping me gain insight into why I came to this earth, which inspired this book, and teaching me to stop and smell the roses. Lastly, I would like to thank the tens of thousands of patients who have entrusted me with their vision needs over the years; without their input, I would not have the expertise or experience to write this book.

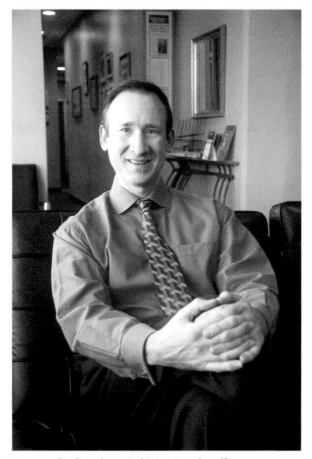

Dr. Dougherty in his Los Angeles office

Seeing Is Believing

Giving thousands of people the gift of sight has been a dream of mine that I've been fortunate to live out. Beyond performing daily surgeries and examining patients, I also travel the world teaching eye surgeons the latest techniques in vision correction.

The field of refractive surgery is an extraordinary and quickly evolving field. Over the years eye care has taken leaps and bounds, but now more than ever patients can achieve the vision they've always "envisioned"—excellent sight with less dependence on glasses and contact lenses. I am thrilled at the progress in my profession, but I have never been more excited than I am now. In addition to my interest in laser vision correction, my current expertise is in the latest frontier of vision correction—lens implants.

The quality of vision with lens implants is superior to all other procedures because it maintains the natural optical system of the eye. I have studied and practiced various surgical techniques, and upon personally assessing a patient's needs, I know what is best for each patient. As I have years of experience in each of the different types of surgery, I am able to recommend what is best for the patient, not necessarily what is easiest for the doctor. I tell each of my patients, "I am treating your eyes as if they were my own." LASIK has helped many, but it is the best option for only about half of vision correction candidates. At moderate to high levels of treatment, LASIK cannot compare with the optical performance of the new lens implants that I have helped develop.

Most new patients hear about me through a personal referral, yet often the first step in the journey to better vision is a visit to my website (www.doughertylaservision.com) to learn about my background and Dougherty Laser Vision's unique breadth of services. On our YouTube site (www.youtube.com/user/doughertylaservision/videos) is a video archive of my latest TV news and reality series appearances and patient testimonials. I have also included dynamic reviews of my various procedures, research activities, and patient testimonials. There's also an overview of the unsurpassed refractive surgery technology employed at Dougherty Laser Vision as well as additional new stories.

My goal is to provide potential patients with educational resources to make a wise decision in protecting one of their most valuable and irreplaceable assets—their eyes.

"One's destination is never a place, but a new way of looking at things."
—Henry Miller

"The way we see the problem is the problem."
—Stephen Covey

"When we change the way we look at things,
the things we look at change."
—Wayne Dyer

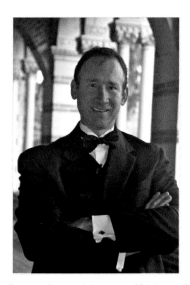

Dr. Dougherty prior to giving one of his invited lectures

My Vision

My dream is to train a national group of vision correction surgeons united under the umbrella of affiliated private practice vision centers delivering the highest quality, most sophisticated eye care available anywhere. Parallel to this, I am developing World Vision Project philanthropic organization that would bring this same level of eye care to impoverished families in the United States and throughout the Third World.

The purpose of this book is twofold. First, I hope to educate people about the superior viability and performance of lens implants; and second, I hope to solicit allies in a worldwide journey: bringing the highest quality vision care to all, in all regions of the world.

3

Why Patients Come to Me

Experience: As one of the most experienced vision surgeons in the world, I have performed over 22,000 laser vision procedures and 8,000 lens procedures since 1993 and have trained thousands of surgeons from all over the world in my techniques. I have given well over one hundred invited lectures and live surgery symposia at universities and eye conferences on six continents, and recently received the prestigious American Academy of Ophthalmology Achievement Award for distinguished service in education to my fellow ophthalmologists. I have published over fifty scientific articles, book chapters, and educational articles in peer-reviewed and trade journals. I am one of a small group of surgeons in the world to have served on the editorial board of the Journal of Refractive Surgery—the international scientific journal for vision correction surgeons published by the American Academy of Ophthalmology. I have been guest editor-in-chief for two of this esteemed organization's publications.

Among Dougherty Laser Vision's proudest accolades are the awards bestowed by two prominent publications: LASIK center of the year by the *Los Angeles Daily News,* and the best LASIK center in Ventura County by the *Ventura County Star* for the last six years in a row.

As one of the most experienced surgeons in the world, I frequently consult with patients from around the globe, often dealing with refractive surgery complications in patients who have had surgery with other surgeons. Many of my colleagues call me the "fix-it" doctor, a moniker I wear with humility.

Training: Unlike most surgeons, who take a weekend course and/or practice refractive surgery part-time, I did a yearlong intensive fellowship in corneal and refractive surgery with Dr. Richard Lindstrom at Phillips Eye Institute in Minneapolis, specializing in all aspects of vision correction surgery.

In addition, unlike most surgeons, my practice is limited to lens and laser-based vision correction surgery.

Technology: Because of my special training, I don't just use available technology; I help to develop it. I have been a principal investigator in multiple Phase III FDA studies and have been involved in the development of three important (or soon to be important) vision correction technologies. The first is the Visian ICL (the lens implant used in the Vista Vision ICL procedure) made by Staar Surgical, Inc.; this is a high-definition alternative to LASIK or for patients who can't have LASIK. The second is the Tetraflex IOL made by Lenstec, Inc., an accommodative IOL (allowing people to see distance and use the natural muscle in the eye to see close) which is likely to change the landscape of modern IOL surgery.

And third, I am proud to be involved in the development of topography-guided LASIK (Customized Aspheric Treatment Zone - CATz made by Nidek, Inc.) which uses 7000 data points as a basis for customized LASIK treatment (compared to 200 data points with current generation custom lasers). This laser is currently used internationally to remedy patients with problems associated with older generation lasers such as night glare and halo, decentered treatments, and poor vision quality.

Dougherty Laser Vision's arsenal of cutting-edge equipment sets my practice apart from other vision surgeons. I have at my disposal multiple excimer laser and keratome technologies, including the Nidek EC-5000 excimer laser, the Visx Star S4 excimer laser, the Alcon Ladarvision excimer laser, and the Nidek MK-2000 microkeratome. The Dougherty center's Ziemer LDV Laser Microkeratome—the new state-of-the-art laser for flap creation, which is the only laser allowing for true "all-laser LASIK" and has replaced the older IntraLase Microkeratome in my practice—is the first in Los Angeles, Ventura, and Santa Barbara counties.

I also offer, and have experience with, every refractive ICL and IOL on the market in the US, including the Staar Visian ICL, the AMO Verisys ICL for moderate and high nearsightedness, the Staar Nanoflex, Lenstec Tetraflex and

Softec HD, Bausch and Lomb Crystalens HD and AO accommodating IOLs, the Alcon Restor, and the AMO Tecnis and Rezoom IOLs for the correction of presbyopia (reading vision). With all of the most modern technology, I am able to tailor the procedure, as well as the equipment, to the individual patient's visual needs.

Caring: A "heart virtue" is the underlying definition of the predominant qualities of each person's soul—that is, who they are essentially as a human being. Each of us is born with unique heart virtues, which follow us for the rest of life, silently defining what is most important to us. I feel that anything that we do in alignment with these heart virtues will give us a great sense of fulfillment and accomplishment.

I once did a personal introspection workshop with my good friend, mentor, and colleague, Greg Mooers, whose most pronounced heart virtue is unquestionably spiritual integrity. Greg is a former artificial intelligence savant who gave his successful company to his employees and joined a monastery for eight years. Upon leaving the monastery, he has gone on to publish and speak extensively about these heart virtues and work as a life coach. In my opinion, Greg and his Bridge 2 Bliss initiative will be the next Tony Robbins in terms of a positive contribution to society.

When I did this dynamic personal research with Greg, I learned that I am committed to connection, fairness, and compassion: These are my deepest heart virtues. By caring for my patients and performing the most delicate eye surgery, I get to put these virtues into action every day.

Connection is a meaningful key in my life because I am fortunate to meet hundreds of patients per month and very quickly establish a deep connection. The thrill of changing people's lives in a positive way never wears off.

Fairness is a quality I developed early on. In my profession, I see that it sets me apart from many others. Rather than coerce patients into unnecessary surgery or perform surgery on borderline candidates, I exercise my fairness virtue by recommending to them exactly what I would recommend doing to my own eyes—nothing more, nothing less.

Compassion is perhaps at the core of my caring. As an eye surgeon, if someone has a less than expected outcome with me or another surgeon, I get to care for that person and do whatever it takes to fix the problem. The caring that I try to give to each patient is influenced by the fact that I had LASIK surgery on my own eyes in January 1997, and I know firsthand the questions, fears, and doubts that most people go through. As one of the first ophthalmologists in the world to have LASIK on his own eyes, I certainly had fears of my own going into the procedure.

As a former patient, I understand the conflicts that most patients go through in undergoing surgery on their own eyes. I treat every pair of eyes like they are my own. I recommend the specific procedure that I would have myself if I were in their situation.

Lastly, I have a handpicked staff that is focused on customer service and delivering the best patient care possible. As an indicator of their trust and faith in my abilities, many of these staff members have undergone refractive surgery by me.

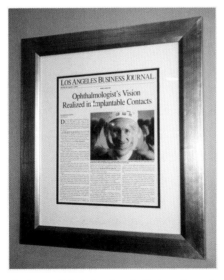

Feature article in *Los Angeles Business Journal*

4

My Clientele: Celebrities, Boomers, and People Just Like You

Vision correction via refractive surgery is always elective, meaning it's the patient's personal choice rather than being dictated by an urgent medical need. This is why insurance typically does not pay for these vision correction procedures unless a patient has visually significant cataracts. Patients from seventeen to one hundred years of age can have refractive surgery, as long as their glasses prescription is stable.

The reasons for opting for refractive surgery are many and varied. Some patients just dislike or are intolerant of their glasses and/or contacts. Many people have surgery because they do not like how they look in glasses, and/or glasses interfere with their job, or with leisure activities such as sports or swimming. Contact lens intolerance due to dry eyes or allergies is a challenge for some. In fact, the lack of humidity in regions of the United States such as Arizona and California (where my primary offices are located) is a contributing factor to the early popularity of refractive surgery in these regions. However, LASIK and other vision correction surgeries eventually caught on in other regions with greater humidity and a less "outdoor-oriented" lifestyle as well. Other patients who often come in for surgery include police officers, firefighters, or people who want to be hired for jobs where there is a visual requirement. Lastly, some patients simply don't like the hassle of glasses or contacts.

As the baby boomers age, many elect to have surgery for reading ("monovision" LASIK). Eventually, almost all will develop cataracts and choose IOL implantation. Both of these age-related situations are becoming more common in my practice.

On the younger end of the spectrum, I am doing vision correction for more and more actors from Hollywood. I have performed surgery on actor and comedian Dennis Miller, Leighton Meister (star of TV's *Gossip Girl* and the recent movie *The Roommate*), Tommy Flanagan (TV's *Sons of Anarchy* and the movies *Braveheart* and *Gladiator*), actor/comedian T.J. Miller (star of the recent film *Cloverfield*), Leeza Gibbons (television personality and philanthropist), Josh Henderson (TV's *Desperate Housewives*), Chris Myers (Emmy Award-winning Fox Sports announcer), Hal B. Klein (2008's *Bottle Shock* movie), Chris "The Kid" Reid (comedian, rap musician, star of the *House Party* movie and the *Kid 'n' Play* TV series), Leslie Silva (actress from TV series *CSI: Crime Scene Investigation* and *CSI: Miami*), Sophina Brown (from TV's *Shark* and *Chappelle's Show*), as well as many others.

In addition, all of my friends or family members who were candidates for surgery have come to me for procedures, including my attorney brother and my mother.

"See no evil, hear no evil, taste no evil, touch no evil, and think no evil."
—Anonymous

"Never see where you are, only your goal."
—Anonymous

"Vision is the art of seeing things invisible to others."
—Jonathan Swift

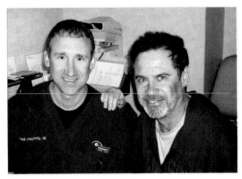

With comedian Dennis Miller

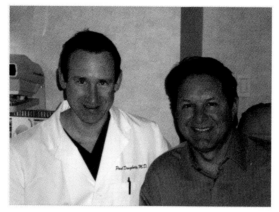

With Chris Myers, Emmy Award-winning FOX sportscaster

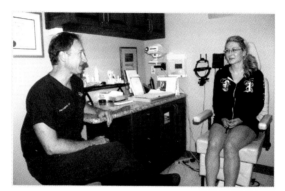

Talking with my patient, *Playboy* Playmate and
radio hostess, Andrea Lowell

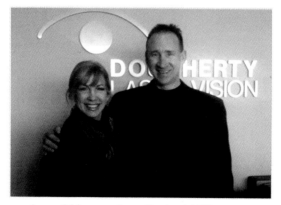

Leeza Gibbons and me after her LASIK surgery

5

My Early Years

The idea of serving others is really the vision behind my vision. Ironically, the story of my physical vision actually began with its partial loss. When I was in high school my eyesight began to blur; I was subsequently diagnosed with nearsightedness and wore corrective glasses and contact lens. Naturally I endured the taunts of my peers, never dreaming that one day I would be able to help others see, both through philanthropy and via developing new vision technologies. My nearsightedness has been only a physical limitation, and I have trusted my heart virtues to guide my compassionate endeavors.

I grew up in early 1970s in a middle-class Pennsylvania family, but because it was such a large brood, I had to fight for the last piece of food and to get the best seat in the car. Probably I should have grown up to be a very selfish person. Yet, if I can be at all objective about myself, I sincerely believe that I am a very caring person. My mother likes to tell the story of when I was three years old, and Santa Claus called me up to give me a present at a church Christmas party. Before accepting it, I insisted that Santa give my four-year-old brother a gift before accepting mine, an unexpected act that warmed my mother's heart and, I'd like to think, set a benevolent tone for my life.

I was the second of five children and grew up in a small rural community. It was a very different life than most of us now live in our rushed super-urban environments. As children, we roamed the neighborhood and surrounding woods without supervision. In a town of 6,000 people, everyone pretty much knew everyone. When someone did anything, good or bad, it spread through the grapevine with astounding speed. Because television reception was limited to a few "snowy" network channels, and personal electronic devices did not exist, we were perfectly happy to entertain ourselves.

My days were mostly filled with sports, ever in the midst of my brothers, my only sister, and the neighborhood kids. I was into every new hobby I could find including sports, hiking, and fantasy baseball. My father, an oral surgeon, spent most of his time working with his patients or reading, and my mom's days were filled with a hundred household chores. From an early age, I learned to be self-sufficient and recognized the importance of taking care of myself both physically and emotionally. Each of us kids helped share family chores, including mowing the lawn in summer, raking leaves in fall, and shoveling snow in winter.

To earn money for college and medical school, I sold Jack & Jill ice cream and fresh pretzels in the rough neighborhoods of northeast Philadelphia. As an independent contractor who rented a truck and bought the ice cream in advance, my money was lost unless I worked hard. Fifteen-hour days were the norm. Once a thief came up to the truck and asked me how much money I had and told me that he had a gun. I convinced him that robbing me was not in his best interest since I did not have that much money. Scowling in disbelief at my candor, the thief bolted away. A narrow escape for this young entrepreneur—*whew!*

The beloved American artist Norman Rockwell was once asked if he had any advice for today's young people. He replied, "Well, the first thing I'd do is to get myself born in a small town in New Hampshire, and after that, things would pretty much take care of themselves." That's basically what happened to me in Pennsylvania.

Whatever compassion and acceptance of others I learned, I learned it the hard way—for I was frequently on the receiving end of very non-compassionate teasing. In my family of four boys and one girl, I was the skinniest. I was so painfully thin, in fact, that my siblings and the neighborhood kids called me "Bones"! When we played tackle football or wrestled in the family room, I always bore the brunt of my older brothers' merciless roughhousing.

Also, because my mother is Croatian, I looked different than all of the other kids, and was frequently mistaken for having Asian ancestry. To my

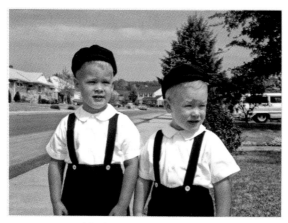

My older brother Jack and me, 1965

embarrassment, my nickname in junior high was "Chink" (needless to say, political correctness was unheard of then). I laughed it off, but inside it hurt.

Looking back, I now see how experiences like these were part of my process of learning compassion—by feeling the pain of a lack of compassion from others. Overcoming deficits are often how we develop strengths. My years of helping with bake sales at the local church, pancake breakfasts for the Kiwanis Club, and delivering food to the elderly and the needy as a Boy Scout were all part of my training to eventually work in the service industry.

Unquestionably, one of the biggest influences on my early life was the Boy Scouts. My scoutmaster, Ken Jones, was truly an amazing person. His daughter was severely mentally retarded with Down syndrome, and I could not understand how this man who had such tragedy in his own life could give so much to others. I was one of the scouts that Ken mentored to become an Eagle Scout, the organization's highest rank. When he was not working or spending time with his daughter and wife, he spent time with scouts like me, helping us grow up to be responsible, hardworking, and caring people. I think my interest in others stemmed from Ken and his daughter—who was not a source of pain and sadness, but rather, despite her disability, a source of pride and joy.

My parents both worked in health care—my father was an oral surgeon and my mother was a public health nurse. I saw the satisfaction that they got from caring for people. It was so inspiring to me to see how they put others' needs in front of their own. I remember one day my father was outside having fun with us kids on a gorgeous fall afternoon. My mother yelled to him that one of his patients was on the phone with a problem. Next thing I know, despite the joyous time he was having with us (which were few and far between, owing to the demands of his career) he left to care for his patient, as if it were an emergency.

With my parents as professional role models, I went to college at the University of Pennsylvania and majored in neuroscience with the intention of going to medical school. My major was Biologic Basis of Behavior, which incorporated neuroscience, psychology, and anthropology. It focused on the interconnection between mind and brain. At the time, I did not understand the intricate interconnection between the mind, the body, and the spirit. All I knew was that I wanted to learn what we humans were all about.

Later in life, when I attended Greg Mooers' personal introspection workshop to discover what means the most to each individual, I discovered that I was committed to connection with others through fairness and compassion. This is my most basic drive in life. Only after this particular workshop did I begin to realize why I had chosen my particular academic path: to learn more about other humans so that I could connect with them.

I moved to Los Angeles when I was luckily accepted at the UCLA School of Medicine as an out-of-state student. (Who could give up the opportunity to allow the taxpayers of California to subsidize my education at such a world-class medical institution?) It was there that I had a major lesson in humility. As first-year medical students, we were to dissect a human cadaver. The first day shocked me—the smell of formaldehyde and the sight of a healthy looking (except for his ghastly color) fifty-year-old gentleman underneath the lid of the cadaver box. After getting over the initial repugnance at seeing and smelling the cadaver, I got to know my colleagues. One was a former female attorney in her mid-forties who seemed very nervous, and kept saying that she did not belong with the rest of us because we were so smart.

A few weeks into the semester, we had our first anatomy test. Because I had been gifted with a photographic memory, I had always done well on tests. The day after the test, as we were dissecting our cadaver, the erstwhile attorney said to me, "I failed the test, and can you believe it, someone actually got 100 percent?!" I sheepishly said, "That was me." She abruptly turned on her heels and left the room. I never saw her again, and she resigned from medical school that day. From that day forward, I have tried to practice a little humility.

Because of my background in neuroscience, and my belief (at the time) that the brain was the source of life, I thought I wanted to be a neurologist or neurosurgeon. I began to take electives in neurology and neurosurgery. While the subjects were fascinating, I was frustrated with how much we physicians did not know about the nervous system, and how little we could do for patients with irreversible neurologic disease, such as head trauma, stroke, Parkinson's disease, and multiple sclerosis. I felt that I had come to this earth to do something - not just classifying diseases we could do nothing about.

My decision to go into ophthalmology was made at three a.m. in the neurosurgery operating room at UCLA Medical Center, while I was assisting in removing a subdural hematoma from a patient who had been in a serious motorcycle accident without a helmet. As I was assisting with the procedure, I realized that this young man was either about to die or remain in a permanent vegetative state. For some strange reason, I found myself hoping that the patient would at least be able to see. Then it dawned on me ... To *see*! That's what I wanted: to pursue a life in *ophthalmology*.

Within days, I was filling out an application for ophthalmology residency training and had my residency interview with Dr. Straatsma, chairman and founder of the Jules Stein Eye Institute. He asked me what made me think I would be a good surgeon. Even though he was such a distinguished teacher and surgeon, I boldly informed him that I had excellent hand-eye coordination because I was an excellent ping-pong and pinball machine player. I couldn't believe the naiveté of what I had just said, and I was so relieved when he hired me!

At UCLA's Jules Stein Eye Institute, I was exposed to all aspects of ophthalmology. However, what excited me most was a sub-specialty that was just in its formative stages—refractive surgery (vision correction surgery). I was so excited about this young field because, as I mentioned earlier, I had been wearing contacts and glasses for nearsightedness since high school. I instantly knew that this is what I wanted to do with my life—help people get the surgery that I knew was going to change my own life.

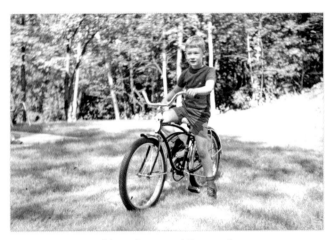

Me and my new bike, age 5

In the early 1990s, LASIK (laser-assisted in situ keratomileusis—essentially lifting a flap and reshaping the cornea with a non-thermal laser) had just been invented and was not yet widely performed. RK surgery (radial keratotomy—flattening the cornea to treat nearsightedness by weakening the peripheral cornea with deep radial cuts made by a diamond knife) was the predominant way to correct vision, even though it was not as accurate or stable as LASIK proved to be. The excimer laser (the part of LASIK that re-shapes the eye for vision) was just in the early study phases when we obtained one at Jules Stein Eye Institute during my last year of residency. Excimer lasers break carbon-carbon bonds in a photochemical, not photothermal, process that allows removal of tissue without creation of heat. Heat creates scarring, which is not good for the clear window we see through, known as the cornea.

That was a turning point. I knew I just had to get involved in this new technology. I approached the cornea fellow and the new refractive surgeon at UCLA, who were also just learning about the mechanics of refractive surgery, to tell them of my interest in the technology. Soon we were meeting to discuss various important issues with this new laser. At the time, not much was understood about why some patients got different results than others. It was felt that the water content of the cornea might vary from patient to patient, and from surgical technique to surgical technique, which could lead to variable results. The three of us came up with a technique to prove it. Lo and behold, we were correct: Wetter corneas responded to treatment at a slower rate. This knowledge is still used in our field today to maximize outcomes in LASIK. I had never written a scientific article before, but I knew that our results were so compelling that I had to let the world know. My passion for surgical vision correction pushed me to put everything I had learned into an article for one of the top peer-reviewed ophthalmologic journals.

The most interesting thing about writing the article was learning about the very specific format and scientific technique it had to incorporate. Today, as an author of scientific articles and editor and reviewer for *The Journal of Refractive Surgery*, I look back on that first scientific article fondly. I published the award-winning research on excimer laser ablation rate and corneal hydration in *The American Journal of Ophthalmology*. It turned out to be one of the pioneering works in the field, and I am still referenced in many current studies. The paper helped lead to standardization of techniques.

With this passion and research background, I was fortunate enough to be selected (out of several hundred applicants) to spend a year of fellowship study with world-renowned Dr. Richard Lindstrom at the Phillips Eye Institute in Minneapolis. Dr. Lindstrom is arguably the most recognized ophthalmologist in the world and was instrumental in introducing LASIK into the United States. It was like a dream to be able to work closely with such a true pioneer and visionary. At first, I was completely in awe of him. When he looked me in the eye and spoke to me as a colleague rather than a lowly trainee, I gained instant respect for him. Beyond his surgical skills, I found the level of trust he had in me amazing. My first day assisting his surgery, he performed the most beautiful corneal transplant I had ever seen. Most surgeons take one to two hours to perform such a surgery. He did this very complex procedure in an astounding twenty minutes.

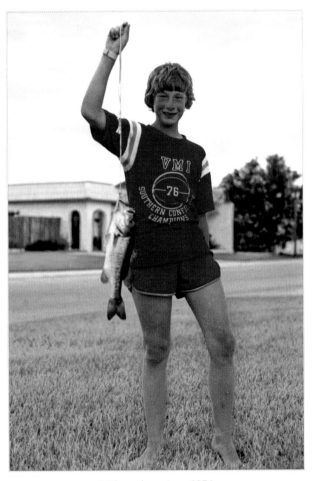

With my bass, June 1976

Then, the next cornea transplant patient arrived in the room—for *me* to operate on! Dr. Lindstrom told me that he would be in the next room performing cataract surgery, and I should call for him if I needed him. In no time, I was performing beautiful transplant surgery thanks to my incredible training, plus the trust he put in me. Of the nearly one hundred transplants that I performed in my fellowship year, I had one case where the patient was seeing 20/30 on the first day—good enough to pass the driver's license test without glasses, which was unheard of with a cornea transplant! Boy, was I proud. (Time for my practice of humility … again!) When my mentor saw this patient with me the next day, he simply said (with classic Minnesota humility and reserve), "Good job."

Dr. Lindstrom's initial trust in me was like a bank account that accrued extraordinary interest as the mentor/pupil bond developed. Once, when I was seeing a Native American patient who had fallen while intoxicated and ruptured the cornea transplant in his only eye, I called Dr. Lindstrom for advice, and he told me, in his characteristic warmhearted, paternal tone: "Do what you were trained to do." I spent the rest of the night fixing this patient's ruptured globe and restoring vision in his only eye. Slowly, but surely, I began to believe in my training and my ping-pong and pinball powers!

Dr. Lindstrom is one of the most talented cataract surgeons in the world. The first case I ever saw him perform was on a patient with multiple risk factors—a dense cataract (cloudy lens of the eye), small pupil, and a finding known as pseudo-exfoliation, which is whitish material in the front of the eye, indicating that the attachments that hold the lens to the eye are very weak. As expected, the surgery was very difficult and a serious complication arose: the loss of vitreous material, which you try to avoid because it increases the rate of retinal swelling and detachment after surgery. In awe as I was of my seemingly infallible new mentor, I could not believe that he had lost vitreous! After the case, he calmly said to me that he felt badly that the patient had suffered this consequence, but that he had done his best under the circumstances, and that she was likely to do well despite the complication.

———

The next day in the clinic, I saw Dr. Lindstrom explain the situation to the patient in the most honest, humble, and compassionate way I had ever seen. It was then and there that I had a clear understanding as to how I was going to practice and perform.

Prior to receiving United States FDA approval, Phillips Eye had the most experience with laser vision correction in the country. I spent a full year working there with Dr. Lindstrom, learning to perform RK, laser vision correction, and cornea transplants. I performed my first laser vision correction procedure under his tutelage in 1993, two years prior to the FDA approval of the excimer laser for LASIK in the United States. Since then, my career has been focused on performing surgeries and developing techniques and technology for the surgical correction of vision.

"That only which we have within can we see without."
—Ralph Waldo Emerson

"What we see depends mainly on what we look for."
—John Lubbock

"Every man takes the limits of his own field of vision
for the limits of the world."
—Arthur Schopenhauer

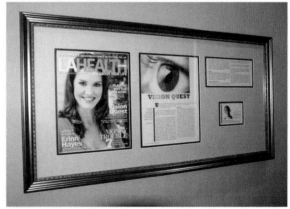

Article on Vision Quest

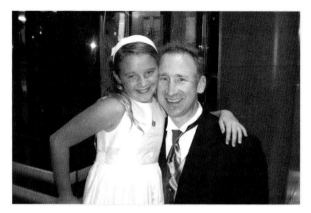

My daughter Abigail and me on a cruise

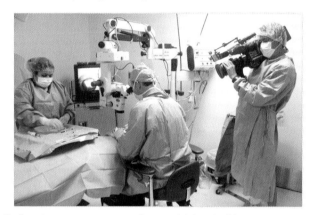

Performing surgery on one of my multiple television appearances

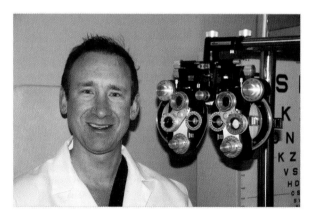

Me in my office

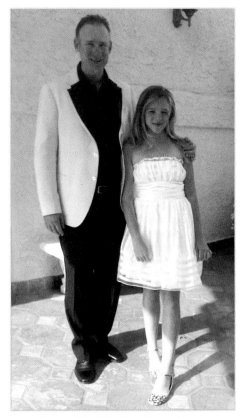

My daughter Abigail and me at home

Why Do People Need Glasses/Contacts?

People need glasses or contacts because of a common problem called refractive error, which blurs vision. There are four different types of refractive error: nearsightedness, farsightedness, astigmatism, and presbyopia. Nearsightedness and farsightedness are always mutually exclusive, but astigmatism and presbyopia may occur alone, with each other, and with nearsightedness or farsightedness. In order to understand refractive error, one needs to think of the eye as acting like a camera.

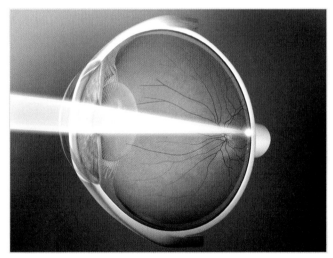

Cross section of an eye that does not need glasses to see. Note that there is a perfect balance between the eye curvature and the length, resulting in perfect focus on the retina. ©2010 Eyemaginations, Inc.

The cornea (the transparent window forming the front of the eye) and the eye's natural lens act like the lens of a camera to focus light onto the retina in the back of the eye. The retina functions like the film of a camera by receiving light images and translating them into electrical impulses that are transmitted to the brain and interpreted as vision. Patients who have no refractive error and do not need glasses or contacts to see perfectly have a perfect balance between the curvature of the front part of the eye (primarily the cornea) and the length of the eye, so that light images focus sharply on the retina. In the normal eye, close images can be focused on the retina by increasing the power of the natural lens through accommodation, which is the ability of the eye to change its focus between distant objects and near objects.

Nearsightedness (myopia) is the most common refractive error, affecting approximately 40% of the population of the United States. Nearsightedness occurs because the eye is too long or the cornea is too steep, resulting in blur (because images are brought into focus in front of the retina). Without corrective lenses, nearsighted people (in medical terminology, myopes) can see things up close but not far away. Myopia is treated surgically by decreasing the focusing power of the eye by flattening the cornea (LASIK/PRK) or by adding a negatively powered lens (ICL/IOL).

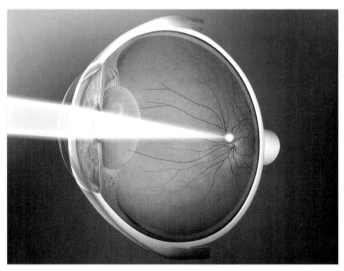

Cross section of a myopic (nearsighted) eye. Note that light is focused in front of the retina, resulting in blur. ©2010 Eyemaginations, Inc.

Farsightedness (hyperopia) is also a common refractive error that requires glasses or contact lenses to correct. Farsightedness occurs because the eye is too short or the cornea is too flat, resulting in blur (because images are brought into focus behind the retina). When farsighted people have accommodation of their lens during their younger years, they can see up close and distantly without correction. As they age, hyperopes (people who are farsighted) first lose their reading vision (which takes the most accommodation), then their intermediate vision (computer) and, finally, their distance vision, requiring glasses or contacts. Because hyperopes maintain distance vision until they get older, the condition is called "farsightedness."

This familiar term for hyperopia is confusing, however, because hyperopes eventually lose their ability to see distance without glasses as they get older. Younger patients with significant hyperopia require glasses for far and near vision if their level of hyperopia is so high that their accommodative mechanism (zooming power of the natural lens) is not strong enough to compensate. Hyperopia is treated surgically by increasing the focusing power of the eye by steepening the cornea (LASIK/PRK) or adding a positively powered lens (ICL/IOL).

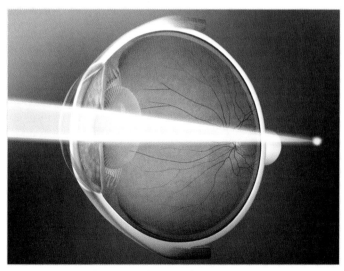

Cross section of a hyperopic (farsighted) eye. Note that light is focused behind the retina, resulting in blur. ©2010 Eyemaginations, Inc.

Astigmatism is a refractive error that blurs vision at all distances because of two different curvatures of the cornea, causing two different images of light from a single light source, neither of which is in focus on the retina. Astigmatism can occur as an isolated visual challenge or in conjunction with nearsightedness or farsightedness. An eye without astigmatism has the same corneal curvature in each direction; to visualize this, think of a non-astigmatic cornea looking like a basketball cut in half. In contrast, an astigmatic cornea is shaped more like a football cut in half, with one direction steep, the other flat. Astigmatism is treated surgically by steepening the cornea in the flat axis and/or flattening the cornea in the steep axis (LASIK/PRK) or adding a lens that is positively powered in the flat axis (ICL/IOL).

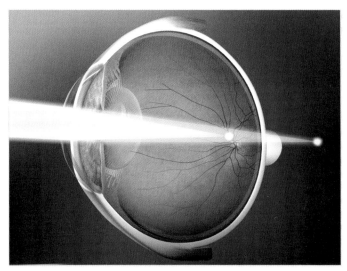

Light in astigmatic eye is focused at two different points from two different corneal curvatures, resulting in blur. ©2010 Eyemaginations, Inc.

Presbyopia is a refractive error that eventually plagues every human being who lives long enough to experience this age-related loss of zooming (or focusing) power in the lens, requiring reading glasses (for people with no other refractive error) or bifocals (in patients that have nearsightedness, farsightedness, or astigmatism). Presbyopia usually begins between the ages of forty-two to forty-seven because of the loss of accommodation. Eye doctors often joke that there are three facts of life: death, taxes, and presbyopia!

Patients in their fifties, sixties, or seventies who claim that they have never needed glasses for distance or near visual acuity are still presbyopic, but they do not notice it, either because they have natural monovision (one eye set for distance, the other for near), or they have a low degree of nearsightedness in both eyes, which allows them to read; consequently, they have gotten used to the distance blur and do not realize that their distance is not perfect. Presbyopia and the loss of vision with age (due to farsightedness) both occur because of loss of accommodation, but they are distinct entities that are commonly confused.

Presbyopia alone results strictly from the loss of accommodation in an eye that has a perfect balance between the curvature of the cornea and length of the eye and requires glasses for reading only; hyperopia results from an eye that is too short or a cornea that is too flat. In hyperopia, glasses are at first needed for reading (due to presbyopia), but eventually required for distance as well. Presbyopia is treated with reading glasses, monovision LASIK/PRK or ICL or with presbyopic IOLs (accommodative or multi-focal).

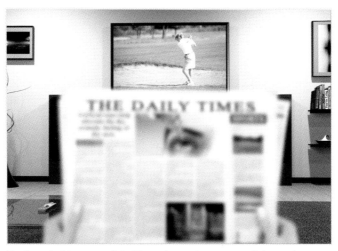

Presbyopia (the age-related loss of zooming power of the eye) creates near blur while distance remains clear. ©2010 Eyemaginations, Inc.

"Your mind is a window through which you see the world."
—Anonymous

"Should one look through a red glass at a white lily,
he would seem to see a red lily."
—M.D. Gabrick

How to Choose
a Vision Correction Surgeon

For the uninitiated, choosing a competent vision correction surgeon can be a daunting task. The critical components for choosing a qualified professional in this field include experience, training, technology, and practice situation. Let us look at each of these qualifications individually.

Experience: It is ideal to choose someone who has performed, at minimum, over a thousand vision correction surgeries. Regrettably, however, many surgeons will not be forthright about their experience. One local surgeon who recently started doing LASIK states that he has performed over 10,000 LASIK procedures—but it turns out these are simple cataract and eye muscle procedures, and this is never disclosed to the patient. A prospective patient needs to ask the surgeon how many times he or she has performed the specific procedure the patient is interested in having done.

Training: The professional ideal is a fellowship-trained corneal and refractive surgeon who has spent a year of additional training (over and above general ophthalmology training) and who does refractive surgery full-time. Most refractive surgeons learn about these procedures in a weekend course; I teach many of these. They then perform surgery as a part-time endeavor, spending the majority of the time dealing with general ophthalmology issues such as basic eye exams, glaucoma, eyelid problems, red eyes, retinal problems, crossed eyes, and children's eye problems, rather than focusing on refractive surgery as a career. As a result, in those unfortunate instances when patients have complications after undergoing surgery with less experienced surgeons, patients are obliged to seek out seasoned, full-time surgeons like myself for "repairs."

For example, I had a patient who had LASIK for monovision (a technique where one eye is set for distance vision and the other is set for reading vision) performed on the wrong eye by a weekend course-trained, part-time LASIK surgeon! The cost to repair the damage was twice what he originally paid with the other surgeon.

Technology: It is important to see a surgeon who has access to—and experience with—the latest technologies, including the latest lens technologies. Most surgeons who perform LASIK or PRK (photorefractive keratectomy, laser eye surgery similar to LASIK) offer this procedure as their only recommendation to the patient. Additionally, many surgeons only have one type of laser (often shared with other surgeons) to perform surgery. In many cases, while LASIK/PRK is possible for the patient, Lens Exchange with an Intraocular Lens (IOL) or the Vista Vision Implantable Contact Lens (ICL) procedure utilizing the Staar Visian Implantable Collamer Lens may be a better alternative for the patient. However, the patient may never know unless a doctor mentions these alternatives.

If the surgeon is either relatively inexperienced or does not offer the alternative lens technologies to the patient, patients will often be encouraged to undergo laser vision correction, even though they would likely do better with a lens implant placed by an experienced surgeon. It is important to look for a surgeon who has access to and experience with multiple types of lasers, because some laser delivery systems work better for certain situations than others. Many surgeons can only afford a single brand of laser and "shoehorn" every patient into this technology. Lastly, many surgeons share lasers, which can be a detriment to overall success, as each laser has its own nuances, advantages, and disadvantages: a distinctive "personality," if you will. I recommend that the patient find a surgeon who has his own lasers with his/her own treatment algorithm or "nomogram" based on the historical outcomes of his/her previous patients.

Practice situation: I recommend choosing a surgeon who is in professional private practice rather than going to a laser company that hires part-time (often weekend course-trained) surgeons. In private practice, the surgeon's focus and commitment is to the patient, not the shareholders. Early in my career, I worked for a vision surgery company whose management answered to its investors. There was both subtle and overt pressure to increase surgical volumes to increase profits. In my experience, laser companies often use non-medical staff that are given bonuses based on productivity and are responsible for convincing patients to book surgery, even if the patient is only a borderline candidate for a particular surgery. This scenario puts even more pressure on the employee surgeon to go along with the treatment plan decided by the laser center staff member, rather than the surgeon, since the surgeon would not evaluate the patient until the day of surgery!

Recently I evaluated a patient who presented for a second opinion prior to surgery, after having been scheduled for LASIK by the staff at a corporate laser center. After my examination, I realized that this patient would have been at very high risk of having a vision-threatening complication from LASIK called ectasia (bulging of the cornea) due to her thin corneas. Instead, I performed the Vista Vision ICL procedure on her with an excellent outcome.

Another shocking problem with choosing a laser company surgeon is that, over the years, many laser companies go bankrupt or shut down if they are not profitable. The latest national laser company to file for bankruptcy protection is TLC Vision (which later became NVision in Southern California). TLC is the company that utilized golfer Tiger Woods as its paid spokesperson. Historically, many laser companies have gone bankrupt or shuttered their doors. In some of these cases, when the patient goes for follow-up with the surgeon, the center is closed, and the patient is forced to find another surgeon—frequently costing the patient more money if additional surgery on their eyes is required and making it difficult or impossible for the new surgeon to have access to critical past medical records.

Lastly, if retreatment or financial issues arise after surgery performed by a corporate laser center, the patient must wade through the bureaucracy of the laser center management (often off-site) for a solution, rather than dealing directly with the surgeon or the staff member who works for him. In a professional private practice, the surgeon is directly accountable to the patient for all medical, financial, and logistical issues and has no account-ability to shareholders in making a decision that is in the best medical interest of the patient.

"You and I do not see things as they are. We see things as we are."
—Herb Cohen

"The only real voyage of discovery consists not in seeing new landscapes but in having new eyes."
—Marcel Proust

"Adventure is merely adversity rightly viewed."
—Richard Byrd

History of Evolving Technology (Glasses, RK, and LASIK)

Refractive error (blurry vision due to an imbalance between the length of the eye and the curvature of the cornea/lens in the front of the eye) comes in four forms, as described earlier: **myopia** (nearsightedness), **hyperopia** (farsightedness), **astigmatism** (or toricity, meaning different corneal curvatures), and **presbyopia** (age-related loss of zooming power of the eye).

Surgery to correct these conditions is known as refractive surgery. Many techniques have been used in the past, and many new techniques are currently being used. The most common problem we treat is myopia, which affects about 40% of the U.S. population. Recently, an article was published in a scientific journal about the myopia "epidemic" in the United States. Since the 1970s, myopia has increased from 25% of the population to over 40%, likely due to the effect of computers and hand-held devices on the development of the eye. These conditions have been treated with glasses for the last few hundred years, and with contact lenses since the 1940s.

In Japan, Dr. Tsutomu Sato first performed "Internal Radial Keratotomy (RK)" for nearsighted patients in the 1940s by using a knife to make slits within the cornea in order to weaken and flatten it. This initially worked well, but most patients ended up needing a corneal transplant due to damage to cells on the inside of the cornea that keep it clear. In Russia in the 1970s, Dr. Svyatoslav Fyodorov popularized RK performed on the outside of the cornea. He is well known for performing this surgery with colleagues on a rotating operating table with each surgeon performing a different task.

RK surgery worked well for mild nearsightedness, and was brought to the United States in the early 1980s. Hundreds of thousands of procedures were performed with good results. The problem with RK was that the higher the prescription, the poorer the accuracy of the procedure. Also, after about a decade of tracking patients, it became evident that about 40-50% of those having the procedure would not have a stable result and become farsighted instead of nearsighted, requiring glasses or contacts again. Many of these patients are now requiring laser or lens surgery in order to see better without glasses.

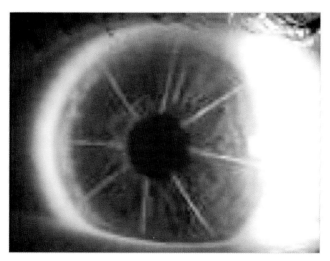

An eye that has undergone 8-cut Radial Keratotomy (RK).
Courtesy of Kent Wellish, MD.

As an alternative to RK, the excimer laser was developed in the late 1980s to treat refractive error by the cool sculpting of the corneal tissue, rather than making cuts to weaken the cornea. In 1987, this laser was first used on the surface of the human cornea after removing the surface cells in a procedure called PRK (photorefractive keratectomy). PRK was more accurate and stable then RK, but was somewhat uncomfortable and associated with blurry vision for a few weeks afterward while the surface cells re-grew over the eye. PRK (flapless LASIK) is still used today for patients who cannot have LASIK because of thin or abnormally shaped corneas. The FDA approved PRK for use in the United States in 1995.

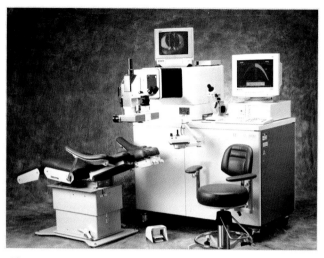

The excimer laser, which is used to re-shape the eye, as part of the LASIK procedure. Courtesy of Nidek, Inc.

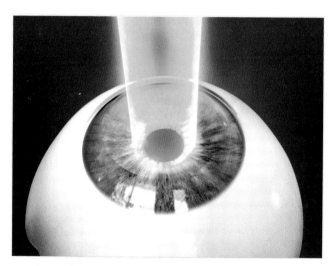

PRK—photorefractive keratectomy. The cool excimer laser is used to reshape the cornea after removing the surface cells. ©2010 Eyemaginations, Inc.

In 1991, a microkeratome (essentially a "planing instrument") was used to create a corneal flap and the excimer laser was used to sculpt corneal tissue under the flap in a procedure called LASIK (laser-assisted in situ keratomileusis). The surface cells of the cornea are left intact in LASIK; therefore the vision returns within a few hours with minimal or no discomfort. As LASIK was more patient-friendly than PRK, it became the procedure of choice for getting people out of glasses. LASIK has become extremely popular, and over seven million procedures have been performed in the United States alone. Doctors began performing LASIK in this country in the mid-1990s as an "off-label (not officially FDA approved) procedure" soon after PRK was approved in 1995. The FDA officially approved LASIK for use in the United States in 1999. Since it was originally developed, some minor modifications of the excimer laser and keratome technology have improved the safety and accuracy of LASIK.

Just as Kleenex is synonymous with a facial tissue, LASIK has become so popular that it has become the generic name most patients use for all forms of refractive surgery, not just LASIK. Both the surgeons and the ophthalmic industry find themselves heavily financially vested in LASIK as the predominant form of refractive surgery. Hence, many surgeons promote LASIK as the best and only way to perform vision correction surgery, even though lens implants may be a better option for some patients.

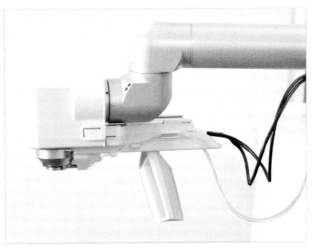

The Ziemer LDV laser keratome: the instrument of choice in creating a flap for LASIK. Courtesy of ZiemerGroup, Inc.

At low degrees of nearsightedness and farsightedness, and for simple presbyopia, LASIK is safe, effective, and has a high degree of patient satisfaction. For these types of vision problems, LASIK will likely be the procedure of choice for the rest of my career.

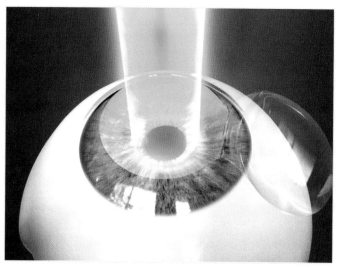

LASIK—the flap and zap procedure. ©2010 Eyemaginations, Inc.

In recent years, some patients have developed a problem following LASIK surgery called ectasia, which is a steepening and thinning of the cornea that blurs vision. Identifying the risk factors for developing this rare problem (such as treatments for high myopia, or thin or irregular corneas) has resulted in refractive surgeons moving away from LASIK in some cases and recommending PRK or lens implants.

The Visian ICL is the most common lens implant used to treat nearsightedness. It is a plastic lens placed in the eye in front of the natural lens. The Visian ICL has been implanted since 1991, and the FDA approved it in the United States in 2005. Originally, it was used only for patients who could not have LASIK because of high corrections or thin corneas. The Vista Vision ICL procedure is my unique way of implanting the Visian ICL. Of late, in my practice, the Vista Vision ICL is replacing LASIK in many cases of moderate and high levels of nearsightedness because the ICL provides the patient with a clearer, higher quality of vision with greater predictability.

The other lens procedure that is used sometimes in lieu of LASIK is refractive lens exchange: cataract surgery with an intraocular lens (IOL) implantation used to get people out of glasses. Typically, this surgery is used for patients

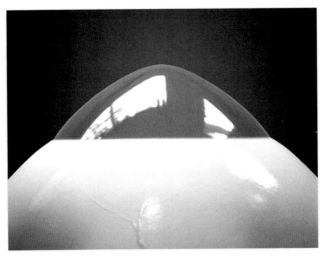

Ectasia—progressive steepening and thinning of the cornea that may rarely occur after LASIK. ©2010 Eyemaginations, Inc.

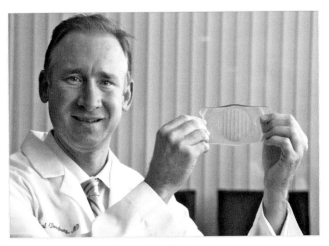

An oversize model of the Vista Vision ICL

over age forty-five that have very high prescriptions or have early cataracts (cloudiness of the natural lens of the eye). In this procedure, the natural lens is broken up and removed with ultrasound and replaced with an IOL, with a focal power customized to the eye. Some newer IOLs have been developed to provide reading vision in addition to distance vision.

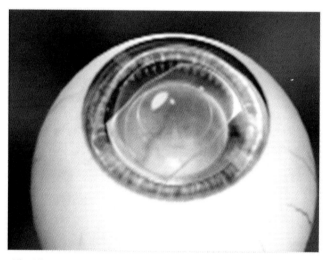

The Vista Vision ICL in the eye, where it sits behind the iris in front of the natural lens. Courtesy of Staar Surgical, Inc.

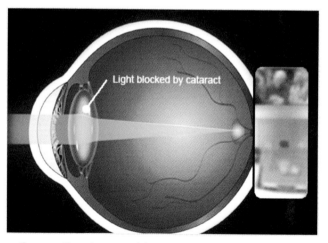

Cross section of an eye with a cataract—age-related cloudiness in the natural lens of the eye. ©2010 Eyemaginations, Inc.

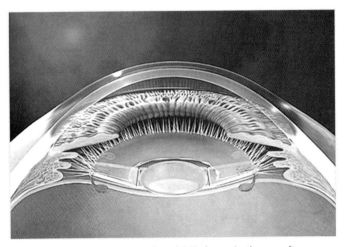

An Intraocular Lens Implant (IOL) shown in the eye after
the cataract is removed. ©2010 Eyemaginations, Inc.

Looking to the future, LASIK and PRK will still be the predominant method
of correcting low degrees of prescription. While there could be some minor
improvements in the laser delivery systems and the microkeratome, the procedure is currently so effective that it will likely not change significantly.

What will change is that lenses (like the Vista Vision ICL and the IOL)
will be performed more commonly because they tend to give better vision
quality than lasers. This is because unlike lasers—which change the optical
properties of the cornea—lens-based procedures do not. These lenses are
additive to the eye (not subtractive; i.e., tissue removing, like laser corrections)
and have the potential to optically correct reading vision at the same time,
something that is not, nor will be in the foreseeable future, feasible with the
lasers. The current generation of lenses have some ability to return reading
vision in the eye of a patient over forty-five years of age, but in the future,
we may have lenses that more closely mimic the natural flexion of the lens,
comparable to when patients were in their twenties.

*"Your vision will become clear when you look into your heart. Who
looks outside, dreams. Who looks inside, awakens."*
—*Carl Jung*

*"The most pathetic person in the world
is someone who has sight but has no vision."*
—*Helen Keller*

"Where there is no vision, the people perish."
—*Proverbs 29:18*

9

Am I a Candidate for Refractive Surgery?

If you wear (or need to wear) glasses and/or contacts to see well and don't like wearing them, you are likely a good candidate for refractive surgery. You should be well informed and willing to take the small risk that is implicit in every surgery. Typically, I operate on people over seventeen or eighteen years of age whose prescription is relatively stable because vision continues to change throughout childhood.

However, we will occasionally perform vision correction surgery on children in unique circumstances. Case in point, I recently had a seven-year-old patient who had high nearsightedness in one eye and was intolerant of contact lenses. Glasses were not an option because of the disparity in power and the resultant magnification difference between the two eyes. She had developed "lazy eye" (an eye that looks normal but cannot see 20/20, even with glasses), with poor vision in this eye due to non-use from the nearsightedness (anisometropic amblyopia). I performed the Vista Vision ICL procedure and astigmatism surgery on this patient in the summer of 2008. Had surgery not been performed, she would have remained blind in this eye for the rest of her life. (For more information on this surgery, see the Associated Press news story and the segment from CBS TV's *The Early Show*, available on my website and YouTube channel, respectively.)

There are a few ophthalmic and medical conditions that can be relative contraindications for refractive surgery. The most common eye condition that precludes laser vision surgery is keratoconus, a disease that involves a progressive steepening and thinning of the cornea, which occurs in approximately one in 2,000 people. There is some genetic predisposition to this

45

disease, so we are always more careful in patients who have a family history of keratoconus or corneal transplantation.

Keratoconics typically have nearsightedness with astigmatism. Early in the disease, they can correct their vision with glasses or soft contacts. As the disease progresses (usually in one's teenage years or twenties), rigid gas permeable lenses or a corneal transplant may be required to see well. Not every patient with keratoconus will eventually require transplantation, however. LASIK makes keratoconus progress; therefore patients with keratoconus should absolutely not have this procedure. PRK may be considered in early cases, since many surgeons believe that removing a little surface corneal tissue does not cause destabilization of the cornea. PRK, however, will not treat any irregularity of the cornea that may be caused by keratoconus. There are many patients that have corneal topography maps that are slightly suspicious for keratoconus (forme-fruste keratoconus) but have no other signs of the disease. These patients (particularly those over age thirty who have shown no progression of the disease) are safe to have PRK with good outcome.

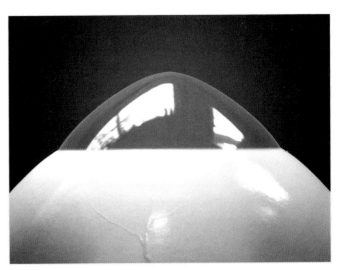

Keratoconus—a progressive steepening and thinning of the cornea caused by a genetic predisposition. ©2010 Eyemaginations, Inc.

Keratoconus may be controlled with two different treatments to stabilize the cornea, including Intacs (small plastic wedges that are inserted in the cornea); and crosslinking of the cornea with riboflavin followed by ultraviolet light that stiffens the weak cornea. Both treatments are not yet approved by the FDA, but have shown great promise at stabilizing this disease. These treatments are available in my practice under a clinical study protocol.

Surgeon friends of mine have also done work overseas using the Toric (astigmatism-treating) ICL to correct vision with patients experiencing early keratoconus. This procedure promises to be extremely viable, since absolutely no corneal tissue is removed, maintaining the stability of the treatment. We hope to have the Toric ICL available in the United States at some point in the near future.

The two general medical conditions that tend to present contraindications in performing refractive surgery (because of poor wound healing) are severe diabetes with retinopathy and severe rheumatoid arthritis. Milder forms of both diseases, however, respond quite nicely to refractive surgery. There is some misconception that refractive surgery is not safe for patients with the wound-healing disease known as keloid formation, various autoimmune diseases, and inactive herpes simplex (cold sore virus). While patients with diagnoses like these were prevented from being enrolled in the various FDA studies of the technologies because of initial concern that these conditions would affect the outcome, both long-term clinical experiences, as well as peer-reviewed publications, show that LASIK and other procedures are safe and effective in these populations. Because patients like these were not enrolled in the FDA studies, such treatment is considered "off-label," that is, not on the FDA labeling guidelines for the technology. If you fall into these special categories your surgeon will ask you sign a special consent form. Most of the things that we do in medicine are off-label (for instance, using aspirin to prevent heart attacks, or using ophthalmic antibiotics, which were approved for bacterial conjunctivitis prior to surgery to prevent infection).

"Leadership is the capacity to translate vision into reality."
—*Warren G. Bennis*

"If what you've been looking for were where you were looking for it,
you'd have probably found it by now."
—*Anonymous*

"Only he who can see the invisible can do the impossible."
—*Frank L. Gaines*

10

Which Options Are Available?
Which Is Best for Me?

There are three main ways to correct refractive error (blurring of the eyes requiring glasses or contacts to see well): laser vision correction (LASIK and PRK), the Vista Vision ICL, and refractive lensectomy (cataract surgery with an intraocular lens, or IOL). All three types of surgery take between three and eight minutes per eye, with both eyes typically receiving surgical correction in the same day. Unfortunately, many surgeons offer laser vision correction as their only vision correction alternative because of lack of experience or familiarity with the other procedures, which may in fact be better suited to the patient.

	Low Myopia	Moderate/High Myopia	Low Hyperopia	Moderate/High Hyperopia	Astigmatism	Presbyopia
Age 18-45	LASIK	ICL or LASIK	LASIK	ICL or LASIK	LASIK	LASIK
Age 45-70	LASIK	ICL or Lensectomy	LASIK or Lensectomy	Lensectomy	LASIK or Lensectomy	LASIK or Lensectomy
Age 70+	LASIK or Lensectomy	Lensectomy	Lensectomy	Lensectomy	Lensectomy	Lensectomy

Chart summarizing the appropriate vision correction procedure for a patient based on age and type of vision problem.

LASIK is the most common surgery performed and can treat nearsightedness, farsightedness, and astigmatism. LASIK (the so-called flap/zap procedure) involves creating a protective flap in the cornea (clear window in the front of the eye) and then gently sculpting the underlying cornea with an excimer laser (cool ultraviolet light laser that removes tissue without scarring). With LASIK, vision returns within a few hours with minimal discomfort.

PRK (photorefractive keratectomy), also known as flapless LASIK, LASEK, or Epi-LASIK, involves removing the surface cells (epithelium) of the eye and then using the excimer laser to gently sculpt the front surface of the cornea to treat the same conditions as LASIK. Because the surface cells are removed and take time to heal in PRK, vision is blurry for the first week or two and continues to improve over the first three months after the procedure. Patients may experience burning, stinging, or discomfort in the first few days after PRK. Typically, patients prefer to have LASIK, and only have PRK when recommended by the surgeon because of thin corneas, irregular corneal shape, or severe dry eyes. Costs range from $1500 to $3000 per eye for laser vision correction.

The Vista Vision ICL procedure is an alternative to laser vision correction for nearsightedness, where an implant is placed in the eye in front of the natural lens through a tiny opening in the outside of the cornea. Surgery is performed on both eyes on the same day. Vision returns immediately, but may remain blurry for the first few days. Discomfort is minimal. The ICL treats nearsightedness at ranges equivalent to LASIK as well as for patients who have a prescription too high for LASIK.

Refractive lensectomy involves removing the natural lens and replacing it with an IOL to treat nearsightedness, farsightedness, and/or astigmatism. Surgery takes approximately five minutes per eye and visual improvement is achieved in hours to days with minimal discomfort. In addition to treating refractive error, there are IOLs available which allow reading vision at the same time (presbyopic IOLs). There are two types of presbyopic IOLs— accommodative (near-enhanced) and multi-focal.

With respect to near-enhancing (accommodative) IOLs, there are multiple types available in the United States. However, the only lens that currently has FDA labeling for accommodation is the Crystalens, which gives excellent distance vision and also has hinges, which allow the lens to flex through contraction of the ciliary muscle in the eye to give better intermediate and reading vision.

There are two other lenses on the market that give excellent distance vision while enhancing near vision, possibly through an accommodative mechanism—the Staar Nanoflex and the Lenstec Softec HD. The Nanoflex works best for patients who are nearsighted, and the Softec HD works best for farsighted patients.

While the Nanoflex and Softec HD lenses are not specifically labeled by the FDA for enhanced near vision, they are more effective, in my hands, than the Crystalens and do not have the potential problems created by the Crystalens, such as Z-syndrome (abnormal bending of the Crystalens at its hinges during the healing process) or night glare from the small 5 mm optic of the Crystalens.

Multi-focal lenses (Restor and Tecnis) act by differentially bending light rays so that some are focused for near vision, others for distance in the same eye. Multi-focal IOLs are the most effective lenses on the market to completely eliminate distance and near glasses (unless the patient tolerates monovision, in which case near-enhanced IOLs with some monovision are also very effective for both distance and near vision without glasses). Restor works best for reading at about 15-21" and works well for intermediate vision (computer) but has the downside of losing some reading effect in low light conditions.

Tecnis, on the other hand, works best for people who like to read or do near activities much closer (12-16"). Tecnis is my preferred lens for patients whose employment requires a very close focal point, like nail technicians or jewelers. Tecnis allows for reading in low light situations but has the downside of some intermediate (computer) blur, requiring the patient to get closer to the computer screen to see well.

Both Restor and Tecnis, because of the multi-focal optics, have the potential downside of causing halos around lights, particularly in low light conditions like night driving. For the vast majority of patients, this symptom is minor, improves with time, and is well worth the trade-off to achieve excellent reading vision without glasses. I do not recommend multi-focal IOLs to patients who do a lot of night driving or might be bothered by nighttime halo.

In deciding on a multi-focal lens versus a near-enhancing lens, the choice is dependent upon your own visual needs. For patients who place more importance on eliminating the need for reading glasses, a multi-focal lens like the Tecnis or Restor is more appropriate. For patients who place more importance on crisp vision in low light conditions, but are comfortable with at least part-time reading glasses, a near enhanced lens like Nanoflex or Softec HD would be more appropriate. The only way to confidently eliminate reading glasses with a near-enhanced lens is by employing monovision. If a patient tolerates monovision, I favor monovision with a near-enhanced lens over a multi-focal lens, due to the lack of halos. Unfortunately, as will be discussed, not everyone tolerates monovision.

Deciding which surgery best suits each patient is a complex process based on the experienced surgeon's determination of the patient's prescription, age, occupation, hobbies, and driving habits, all of which determine the patient's unique visual needs.

LASIK is the most common surgery performed in the United States, and represents about 70% of my surgical vision correction practice. LASIK may be safely used for patients from one to eight diopters (a measure of lens power) of nearsightedness, one to three diopters of farsightedness, and one to six diopters of astigmatism. Because of more discomfort and slower vision recovery, PRK (flapless LASIK, LASEK, or Epi-LASIK) is used only when LASIK is not safe because of thin corneas, irregular corneas, or severe dry eye.

In summary, laser vision correction (LASIK/PRK) is typically used for most patients with lower levels of nearsightedness and farsightedness as well as astigmatism, because it is safe, effective, quick, and minimally invasive. The main downsides to laser vision correction are the potential for development of dry eyes or low-light vision symptoms like glare and halo. Thankfully, both are treatable, and tend to diminish with time.

The Vista Vision Implantable Contact Lens (ICL) is approved to treat nearsightedness from three to twenty diopters. The lens is permanent and is self-cleaning. This lens is made of a material called collamer, which is a plastic and protein co-polymer. Collamer is one of the most biocompatible materials and has some of the best optical qualities of any intra-ocular lens material used in ophthalmology. Unlike other materials, collamer is coated after being placed inside the eye by a natural protein called fibronectin. Because of this, the material is looked at by the body's immune system as an organic component, thereby preventing rejection.

As of today, the ICL is more of a niche product used by a minority of surgeons to treat patients outside the range of LASIK. In the United States, there are only about eight hundred surgeons trained to perform the ICL procedure, but the majority of these surgeons do not offer this technology in the normal course of their practice. This is due to their lack of familiarity/skill with this newer, more surgically demanding procedure, as well as the very small size and lack of marketing by the company that owns this revolutionary technology.

For moderate and high nearsightedness, the advantages of ICL over LASIK include better vision quality, reversibility, and a lower incidence of night vision problems and dry eye. Multiple studies have shown the superiority of the ICL over LASIK and PRK for moderate and high nearsightedness in terms of safety, efficacy, predictability, and stability of the vision after surgery.

Multiple studies have found better contrast sensitivity (vision quality) in ICL than in LASIK. This is because in LASIK, the front surface of the eye is altered with the laser in order to change its shape, resulting in alterations in vision. For low degrees of treatment, these alterations are of no significance, making LASIK a wonderful option. At higher levels of treatment with LASIK, however, these changes in the cornea can result in decreased visual quality and night vision problems like glare and halo. With the Vista Vision ICL, the natural shape of the front of the eye is maintained, resulting in natural "high definition" vision, the way Mother Nature intended. Think of the beauty of a man-made lake (like the man-made corneal surface in LASIK) versus the beauty of a natural lake (like the natural corneal surface in ICL).

Unlike LASIK, the ICL is an additive procedure that can be reversed easily if patients are unhappy with their vision (which has never happened in my practice), or a new vision correction technology is developed that would offer the patient a tangible advantage.

Common side effects of LASIK are not a common occurrence with ICL. ICL patients do not suffer from post-op dry eye like LASIK patients. ICL patients rarely complain of night vision symptoms like LASIK patients, because the cornea essentially remains untouched with ICL surgery. In addition, unlike LASIK, the ICL has an ultraviolent blocking chromophore in the lens material that acts to minimize ultraviolet (UV) exposure to the eye, which can contribute to cataracts and macular degeneration.

The ICL is a permanent lens implant allowing for a lifetime of vision. Any patient, with or without refractive eye surgery, who lives to be old enough, will eventually develop cataracts. At that time, the ICL is easily removed from the eye in a ten-second maneuver, and routine cataract surgery with IOL implantation is performed. When a patient develops a cataract, it is easier to perform accurate IOL calculations in an eye that has undergone ICL, rather than an eye that has had LASIK. Since the corneal curvature is disturbed by LASIK, it is more difficult to precisely measure the true corneal curvature, which is imperative for accurate IOL calculations. On the other hand, an ICL has a virgin central cornea, just as if no surgery had ever been performed on the eye, and IOL calculations are very precise.

Because of the limited thickness of the cornea, LASIK/PRK is only effective up to eight to ten diopters of nearsightedness. Beyond that, ICL is the only option. Traditionally, when the ICL was first approved, this procedure was performed only for high myopes that could not have LASIK. Now, because of the high-definition vision, we offer it to all nearsighted patients over five diopters of nearsightedness, and any patient over three diopters of nearsightedness who has to have PRK because of an abnormal cornea, since ICL gives faster recovery of vision with less discomfort than PRK. In my practice, many patients who want the best quality vision, especially for higher prescriptions, are choosing the Vista Vision ICL over LASIK. Most surgeons in the United States perform the ICL one eye at a time, which is less convenient for the patient and exposes the patient to the risks (albeit minor) of a second trip to the surgical suite.

Also, because the ICL is implanted in the front of the eye, a small hole (iridotomy) must be placed in the iris (the colored part of the eye) either before the lens implant procedure with a laser or during surgery to prevent high pressure or glaucoma in the eye. Most surgeons do not feel comfortable with a surgical iridotomy, requiring the patient to have laser treatment a week before the lens implant. Most surgeons in the United States are just now learning how to perform the ICL and tend to be very conservative with implantation, requiring four separate surgeries (a laser iridotomy surgery on one eye followed at a later time by lens implantation, then the same sequence of events on the fellow eye at a later time). In my practice, I perform both implants on the same day combined with surgical iridotomy. For this reason, my ICL procedure is just as convenient as LASIK. In our practice this highly customized method of ICL implantation is simply known as the Vista Vision ICL Procedure.

In summary, most low nearsighted patients choose LASIK; moderately nearsighted patients select either LASIK or ICL; and highly nearsighted patients choose ICL. The main downside of the ICL is an increased cost (about 20% to 80% more than LASIK—typically $2500 to $4500 per eye). For those patients who, for whatever reason, do not like the idea of a lens inside the eye, they may opt to undergo laser vision correction.

Lastly, refractive lensectomy/IOL is reserved for patients who are older than forty to forty-five (since younger patients still have zooming of the natural lens that allows for reading) and have either vision that is not as accurately treated by LASIK or an early or advanced cataract (clouding of the natural lens). Patients up to age sixty-five or seventy (if they do not have a cataract) are still eligible for LASIK or ICL, which are both slightly less invasive than lensectomy. Nanoflex, Softec HD, Restore, and Tecnis are my first choices in IOLs in refractive lensectomy.

———

As discussed before, Nanoflex and Softec HD seem to enhance near vision (zooming) while giving high quality distance and intermediate (computer) vision. The main downside to these lenses is that most patients will still have to use at least part-time reading glasses, unless they do monovision. Restore and Tecnis are multi-focal (light-splitting) IOLs that give good reading vision without glasses (eliminating the need for reading glasses 90% of the time in my hands) with good distance and fair intermediate vision. The main downside of these lenses is that some patients will experience halo in low-light conditions such as night driving.

In my practice, I utilize a special questionnaire about activities, occupation, and visual preference to decide which type of IOL to use in eligible patients. The main downside to IOLs is that they are more expensive than LASIK (up to $6000 per eye). However, if the patient has a cataract, insurance will typically pay for the surgery, with the cost of the presbyopic IOL package (which is not paid for by insurance) typically similar in cost to LASIK.

To summarize: LASIK is best for low and moderately nearsighted, farsighted, and astigmatic patients, whereas PRK is primarily for those who can't have LASIK because of the corneal thickness or shape. The Vista Vision ICL is for patients with low to moderate nearsightedness who demand the highest quality vision and can afford to pay a little more than LASIK, or for patients with higher nearsightedness who cannot have LASIK. IOLs are reserved for patients over forty to forty-five who have cataracts or are outside the range of LASIK or ICL.

What Are the Risks/
Side Effects of Surgery?

Other than money, the biggest reasons that most people do not have a vision correction procedure are fear, fear, and fear. Studies show that some people rank the fear of blindness above the fear of death. The reality is that refractive surgery is very safe. In fact, patients have twice the risk of losing their vision or losing their eye with a contact lens. The risk of complete loss of vision or the eye from refractive surgery is 1/1,000,000; the risk from a soft contact lens is 1/600,000, typically from an infection. I have performed over 22,000 laser vision procedures and 8,000 lens procedures, including on all of my friends and family members who were candidates. I have never lost an eye from vision correction surgery.

As discussed earlier, in making the decision to have vision correction surgery, one must also be cognizant of the risks and side effects of more traditional vision correction options, namely glasses and contacts. Most people think that contact lenses are without risk. Statistically, over a lifetime, a soft contact lens wearer has a 2% risk of a vision-threatening infection (corneal ulcer). If the contacts are worn overnight, the risk of a vision-threatening infection increases to 6%. The risk of an infection from LASIK is a one-time risk of 1 in 10,000. The main risk associated with glasses (other than losing them in a car accident, earthquake, or other emergency and not being able to see) is that if the lenses are made from glass, trauma that can create a corneal foreign body, corneal laceration, or ruptured eyeball from the lenses shattering, are all possible. Makes your skin crawl, doesn't it? Allow me to repeat: I have never lost an eye from vision correction surgery.

The wearing of both glasses and contact lenses can create side effects. Contact lenses can irritate, dry out, and worsen allergies. When patients are younger, typically the eyes are moist and contacts are tolerated well. As contact lens wearers (particularly females) age, they tend to develop a dry eye condition that makes contact lenses more difficult or impossible to wear because of poor vision and/or irritation. Also, many patients will develop allergies to the contacts or contact lens solution, making the eyes red, itchy, tired, and blurry.

The worst form of contact-related allergy is called giant papillary conjunctivitis (GPC), in which the patient develops large, irritating bumps under the upper eyelid. In terms of vision, contacts can be associated with blurred or fluctuating vision, especially in the circumstance of dry eyes or allergies. Vision blurs or fluctuates with contacts because of changes in the tear film and movement of the lenses as one blinks. Contact lens-related blurry or fluctuating vision tends to be worse at the end of the day as eyes dry out and become tired. This side effect is typically magnified in patients that wear astigmatic (toric) contacts that can rotate and blur vision every time you blink. Contact lenses (particularly rigid and astigmatic contacts) can also be associated with nighttime and low light vision symptoms such as glare and halo.

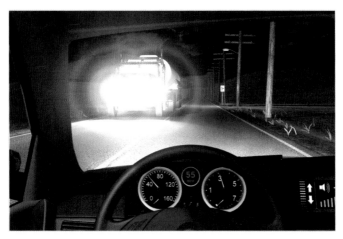

Patient's view of night glare and halo. ©2010 Eyemaginations, Inc.

Glasses can have side effects like diminished peripheral vision and distorted image size, as well as nighttime glare and halos. Such side effects increase as the power of the prescription increases, particularly with astigmatism. This can lead to headache, vertigo, and nausea in some patients. In addition, glasses can be unsatisfactory from an aesthetic standpoint and can be detrimental to certain hobbies or professions because of their bulkiness (think of a swimmer or a photographer trying to use glasses). Glasses can also lead to contact dermatitis (skin allergy) on the nose or ears in some patients. Other patients have difficulty wearing glasses because of a small nasal bridge.

Just like glasses and contacts, every form of refractive surgery has risks and side effects. Fortunately, most risks and/or side effects of refractive surgery are not common, and can be avoided or treated. Please understand that prior to your procedure, you will be asked to sign an informed consent document outlining in detail all of the known potential risks and side effects of each procedure.

If a car salesman were required to spell out the potential risks in buying a car, he would have to present all the data on car accidents and the possibility of actual death. This is not realistic. In my years of eye surgery, my patients are the best testimony to my skill and the wonderful technologies we have available to perfect our vision. Once more, I must emphasize that *I have never lost an eye from vision correction surgery.* I have learned over the course of my career that most of these issues are treatable. The following paragraphs outline the main risks/side effects of each of the major forms of refractive surgery.

LASIK has risks including infection, over- and under-correction, loss of best-corrected vision (BCVA), ectasia, dry eye, night vision problems, and flap complications. In my hands, infection with LASIK occurs about 1/10,000 people. I have seen only two infections after LASIK in my practice. One infection occurred the day after surgery when the patient aggressively dislodged the flap with her finger, and the other LASIK infection occurred spontaneously. Fortunately, both infections were not in the central cornea and were diagnosed early and treated with antibiotic eye drops, and both patients achieved excellent vision without glasses. Over- and under-corrections are easily treated by lifting the previous flap and placing more laser treatment on the cornea.

Vista Vision ICL has risks including infection, cataract, glare and halo, and glaucoma. There have been over 120,000 ICLs implanted in the world with only one documented case of infection, which was diagnosed and treated early with excellent visual outcome. As reported in the FDA study, visually significant cataract occurred only 1% of the time at the seven year follow-up, and was easily and effectively treated with cataract/IOL surgery with good visual outcome. The risk factors for cataract formation with ICL included age over forty and nearsightedness over 13 D (both of which are independent risk factors for cataract formation, even without ICL). Glaucoma (high pressure in the eye) can occur occasionally after ICL and is usually temporary and easily treated with drops. In the FDA study, no patient developed long-term glaucoma. In past years, glaucoma could also be created after the ICL due to an oversize lens. Since the advent of ultrasound technology to measure the sulcus (the area that the ICL is placed in), sizing issues have virtually been

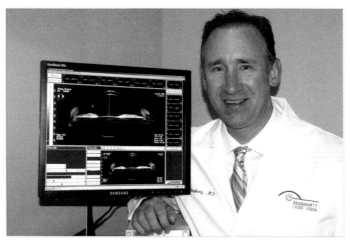

Prior to insertion of the Vista Vision ICL, an ultrasound of the eye (pictured above) is performed to ensure correct sizing of the lens.

eliminated. My practice was instrumental in defining proper sizing of the ICL based on ultrasonic measurement. Unfortunately, because of the prohibitive cost of ultrasound technology, many surgeons performing ICL still determine sizing based on a measurement of the outside of the eye that attempts to predict sulcus size. I am completely confident in this procedure, and ICL is a very solid choice for many patients, with limited risks.

Lensectomy/IOL is a very commonly performed surgery. The risks of refractive lensectomy/IOL are identical to cataract surgery, including infection, bleeding, swelling, retinal detachment, lens dislocation, and glaucoma. Risks are low, and if there are any issues, most of them are readily treatable. Refractive lensectomy/IOL is a definitive procedure, meaning that *the patient will never need cataract surgery*. This is an important factor. As previously discussed, every human being, if he or she lives long enough, will develop cataracts and require cataract surgery. With RL/IOL, the patient exposes themselves to the same risks of surgery that they will eventually need, in exchange for the invaluable benefits of vision correction surgery. Furthermore, because RL/IOL patients are younger and healthier than the average cataract patient, the risk of complications like infection and bleeding are less likely than when the patient is older.

"The word 'insight' means sight from within."
—*Greek scholar*

"Some things have to be believed to be seen."
—*Ralph Hodgson*

"There is a certain sparkle in my eye that I've learned to trust."
—*An old East Indian monk*

12

What about Recovery Time?

Recovery time after vision correction surgery varies based on the proce-dure, but in general, return of full vision is very quick. With LASIK, your vision will be improved almost immediately after surgery, but is still hazy for the first four to six hours, as the swelling of the flap and the dryness of the surface cells dissipate. After this, vision is typically quite good, and most patients are able to drive themselves back to the doctor's office for the post-operative visit and return to work the next day. In terms of discomfort, the eye may feel a little irritated; a feeling like something is in the eye for the first four to six hours after the procedure.

In terms of healing of the cornea, the flap sticks back onto the cornea within sixty seconds. Thus, blinking will not move the flap. This occurs because of the negative stromal swelling pressure of the cornea, which means that the cells on the inside of the cornea (endothelium) pump water from the outside of the cornea to the inside of the eye, which is the mechanism by which the cornea remains clear. This pump sticks the flap back on the underlying corneal stroma, much like putting your hand over the opening of a vacuum cleaner hose while it is turned on. The epithelial incision at the edge of the flap heals within the first three to four hours. Attachments between the cornea and flap (stromal healing) start within the first few weeks and are maximized within six to twelve months. During this period of healing, we advise patients not to rub or put direct pressure on their eyes for the first six months after surgery, with the first two to four weeks being the most critical time period. If pressure is put on the flap that dislocates or wrinkles it, irrigating under the flap and smoothing it easily fixes this.

While quite strong, the interface between the flap and the underlying cornea technically never fully heals after LASIK, which allows us to dissect and relift the flap even years later in order to do an enhancement. Because of this healing pattern, we recommend PRK (flapless LASIK) instead of LASIK for patients who are likely to receive direct blows to the eye (such as professional martial artists or boxers). I performed PRK instead of LASIK on Sebastian "Bas" Rutten, the 2000 Ultimate Fighting Champion (UFC) a few years back for this reason.

Based on healing patterns, the following precautions are recommended for patients after LASIK: No dusty environments nor sweat in the eye for forty-eight hours, and no swimming, hot tubs, nor opening of eyes in the shower for one week after surgery—to prevent infection. No makeup for three days after surgery, and plastic shields must be worn while sleeping for one week after surgery (four weeks if a stomach or side-sleeper) to prevent dislocation of the flap. When removing makeup, the upper and lower lid must be raised away from the eye and pressure put on the underlying orbital bone rather than the eyeball. (As a side note, many people ask me if jumping, running, or flying on an airplane will dislocate the flap. They will not, and are okay immediately after LASIK, providing that no perspiration gets in the eye for forty-eight hours.)

With PRK, vision recovery time is longer than LASIK, and the eye may be more irritated because the surface cells (epithelium) of the eye are removed to perform the procedure and must grow back to provide a clear surface for vision. The blurred vision that occurs after PRK can last for seven to ten days until the epithelium is healed. In the first few days after surgery, the vision may be clearer because the bandage contact lens acts as a refracting surface. By day three or four, the rough epithelial cells have started to move centrally and will blur vision more. The bandage contact lens is typically removed from the eye five to seven days after surgery, but may occasionally be required to be left in place for up to two weeks. The contact both helps speed healing and minimizes discomfort after surgery.

During the initial week of blur, glasses will not help the vision because the prescription has already been treated, and the blur is from rough epithelium. For patients that have PRK on both eyes on the same day (which is

---

preferred by most patients) they are instructed not to drive or return to work for one week. After a week, the vision is typically functional for driving and work, but still fluctuates and is not perfectly clear. It may take anywhere from one to three months for maximal vision while the surface cells are smoothing themselves.

In terms of discomfort, PRK patients may experience anything from no symptoms to more severe pain and light sensitivity. A bandage contact lens, a topical non-steroidal anti-inflammatory (i.e. Advil drop), and a topical anesthetic drop are used to minimize discomfort after the procedure. Because of this protocol, most patients are relatively comfortable after surgery with minimal burning, stinging, tearing, and light sensitivity controlled by ibuprofen (Advil) or acetaminophen (Tylenol) pills. In rare circumstances, particularly if the bandage contact lens inadvertently comes out or is rubbed out, patients can have significant discomfort for a few days requiring a stronger pain medication such as Vicodin or Percocet.

The instructions after PRK are similar to those after LASIK, with the exception of no dust or sweat in the eyes for seven instead of two days. Eye rubbing after the first week is also not as much of an issue as in LASIK. Lastly, PRK patients are instructed to avoid prolonged reading, computer work, or TV watching in the early period after surgery since these activities slow their blink rate and can dry the eye out, prolonging healing.

Vision recovery after the Vista Vision ICL is very similar to LASIK. ICL patients sit up from the procedure table and see better immediately. The vision may be a little hazy or cloudy for one to three days because of dryness on the surface or swelling of the cornea. Most patients are safe to drive and go back to work within twenty-four to forty-eight hours after the procedure. In terms of discomfort, patients may feel a little irritated like something is in the eye for the first twenty-four hours as the tiny corneal incision heals, and they may have dry eye symptoms for the first week or so.

Post-operative restrictions include no swimming or hot tubs for one week and avoiding sweat in the eyes and dusty environments for forty-eight hours to prevent infection. Lifting more than twenty pounds, bending below the waist, and eye rubbing are prohibited for one week to maintain wound stability. Other activities may be enjoyed immediately.

Vision recovery after the lensectomy/IOL varies depending on the patient. Some patients see better immediately; others may take a few days, or occasionally a few weeks depending on the amount of swelling in the cornea. Many patients are safe to drive and return back to work within two to three days after the procedure. In terms of discomfort, just like ICL, patients may feel a little irritated as if something is in the eye for the first twenty-four hours, as the tiny corneal incision heals. They may experience dry eye symptoms for the first week or so.

Post-operative restrictions after lensectomy/IOL are identical to ICL, with most activities allowed almost immediately after surgery.

"Those amazing truths that our descendants will discover are all around us, staring us in the eyes, so to speak; and yet we do not see them."
—*Robert Richet*

"He who knows, tells it not; he who tells, knows it not."
—*Lao-tzu*

What Are the Costs of Vision Correction Surgery? Does Insurance Pay for It?

I f you're considering vision correction surgery, be advised that it is typically an out-of-pocket expense. Fees vary depending on the technology and experience of the surgeon. According to St. Louis, Missouri-based Market Scope (a leading source for data in the ophthalmic marketplace) the average cost in 2007 of LASIK and PRK was $2025 per eye, but can range from $1500 to $3000 per eye. The average price for and ICL and IOL were approximately $4000 per eye. New technology lenses such as presbyopic and toric IOLs cost even more.

Most vision correction practices offer payment plans for the procedure through one or multiple finance companies. Both 0% interest as well as extended payment plans are typically available that can make monthly payments quite affordable for most potential patients.

A helpful mechanism (and tax break) that makes surgery more affordable to many individuals is the FLEX plan, which is essentially *a government-allowed, tax-free medical account that is administered as a benefit through many employers.* The employee simply specifies the year before the plan goes into effect how much money they would like deducted on a monthly, tax-free basis from their paycheck to cover the cost of a medical procedure or product. The employee can undergo surgery at any point during the year, paying for the procedure with the tax-free funds, essentially saving up to 40% of the price of the procedure, depending on their tax bracket.

Unless a patient has a visually significant cataract, which requires a lensectomy/IOL, medical insurance will typically not pay for vision correction procedures because it is considered cosmetic. Under no circumstance (except for a cataract) is an elective vision correction procedure considered medically necessary. I have written many letters to insurance companies to attempt to get LASIK covered as medically necessary when a patient is contact lens-intolerant and/or can't wear glasses (due to allergy to the frames, a small nasal bridge, or high prescription with thick lenses causing distortion). To my knowledge, in no case has medical insurance covered the procedure. The only instance where medical insurance covers LASIK or other vision correction procedures is in situations where they are specifically written into a policy at a higher premium, typically for the benefit of high-level executives of large companies.

If you have an HMO policy, coverage is even less likely than a PPO plan, since HMO payments to your doctor are usually based on a concept known as capitation. Capitation is when the HMO pays the doctor a lump sum of money per month to cover all of the care for a given patient, regardless of how much care the patient requires. If the patient needs surgery or specialty care, the doctor or medical group providing treatment pays the cost. This is why it is typically so difficult to get surgery or a specialty referral in a capitated HMO setting, as the insurance company who owns the HMO policy financially pits the doctor and the patient against one another.

Vision insurance plans also do not typically completely cover LASIK and other vision correction procedures. These plans (i.e., Vision Service Plan (VSP), Davis Vision, or Eyemed) may have negotiated discounts with various surgeons or groups, but rarely directly pay for any portion of the surgery. One notable exception to this is Southern California Edison and certain unions that have plans through vision insurances that pay for up to 90% of vision correction costs. Prospective patients are encouraged to clarify any benefits with the benefits department at their company before undergoing any surgery.

When compared to the costs of contacts, vision correction surgery is less expensive over a patient's lifetime. While a patient might spend $4,000 to $5,000 initially for LASIK, there is no cost for upkeep or maintenance of the results. Contact lens wearers, however, are required to constantly purchase solutions and cleaners for the contacts, as well as change the contacts regularly, with significant cost. From a financial perspective, purchasing vision correction is much like buying a house while paying for contacts is akin to renting one. With vision correction, there is a high initial expense. For example, a $5000 surgery would require a $130/month payment for forty-eight months, and then the vision correction is owned permanently—just like paying a mortgage. Over twenty years, this equates to a cost of $10/month for vision correction. With contacts, there is an average monthly expense of $35 for lenses and solutions, which, like rent, is never ending. Over a twenty-year period, contacts would cost the patient an average of $8400, and would still require an ongoing expenditure. With this analysis, one can easily see that vision correction is a better investment than contact lenses when looked at over a long period of time.

With respect to the price of vision correction, there are many clinics with misleading claims of too-good-to-be-true low prices for LASIK (I have recently seen one as low as $299* per eye). Understand that both the laser used for the treatment as well as the laser keratome that is sometimes used to create the flaps has a royalty fee of hundreds of dollars per eye that needs to be paid to the manufacturer every time the laser is used. Due to the high cost associated with providing LASIK, these discount centers are advertising an unrealistic price and employ a bait-and-switch technique.

Eagle-eyed readers no doubt noticed the asterisk preceding the price in the previous paragraph. This is generally followed by the disclaimer, "certain prescriptions only"—those being typically low prescriptions up to only -0.75 D, which is so low, that most people see very well without glasses and don't really want surgery. Every other type of prescription, including higher degrees of nearsightedness, farsightedness, or any astigmatism, is associated with an up-charge. There is also an up-charge for any newer technology (such as a laser keratome or custom treatment).

Lastly, the patient is nickel-and-dimed by having separate charges for pre-op care, post-op care and retreatments, frequently making the treatments at "discount" centers more expensive than in traditional professional vision correction practices. A few years ago, an exposé on *Dateline NBC* detailed the bait-and-switch tactics used by one of the largest discount eye surgery chains in the United States. The CEO of the company was confronted about the percentage of patients that had surgery performed at the advertised price; he refused to answer the question. The reporter concluded that with the bait-and-switch, *nobody* ever received surgery at the advertised price.

When considering the cost of surgery, the patient also needs to take into account the training and experience of the surgeon. Most surgeons who perform LASIK learn the procedure at a weekend course and perform the surgery part-time for additional income. Many of the discount centers hire these inexperienced, weekend course-trained surgeons to perform these delicate procedures. It goes without saying that lack of experience can lead to a higher rate of complications. When a patient comes to me to fix a problem that has occurred with another surgeon, my fees are higher than if they had had surgery with me in the first place because these cases are typically more complex. (I once had a patient who had surgery with a relatively inexperienced surgeon who advertised low rates. This patient had had the wrong eye set for monovision with LASIK, which required an expensive retreatment by me in both eyes.)

The final issue with discount centers is that the staff members, rather than the surgeon, perform all of the evaluation and testing. Frequently the information that the patient is given about their procedure is more of a sales pitch than evidence-based medical advice. Even more troubling, the patient often does not meet the surgeon until just before surgery, and the surgeon bases his or her technique on the recommendation of the staff. In sharp contrast, in a professional refractive surgery practice, the surgeon is highly involved in patient counseling and surgical planning, rather than delegating this task to employees.

All of these factors must be kept in mind when evaluating the cost of vision correction surgery with a given surgeon. Trusting your eyes to a cut-rate or fly-by-night vision center can have financial repercussions at the very least, and potentially life-altering consequences if your surgeon is inadequately trained or you receive questionable pre-op counsel.

14

What about Near Vision Correction?

Despite a common misconception, all three types of surgery (LASIK/PRK, ICL, and lensectomy IOL) can be performed in a way that maintains or creates reading vision for patients over age forty. This is done with a technique called monovision (blended vision), where one eye is corrected (or left untouched) as a distance eye and the other eye is corrected (or left untouched) as a reading eye.

In cases where patients have good distance vision in both eyes, but have lost their reading vision, one eye can be steepened (usually with LASIK or PRK) to make it slightly nearsighted, and the other eye is left untouched. Typically everyone has a "dominant" or master eye. When we set the eyes for monovision, the dominant eye is set for distance and the non-dominant eye is set for near. While the majority of patients are right eye dominant, you can identify your dominant eye by asking yourself: Which eye would you hold a camera up to? The eye you would choose is your dominant eye.

The ability to "accept" monovision is a brain phenomenon. The brain pays attention to the distance eye for distance tasks and the near eye for near tasks. The main benefit of monovision is the ability to see distance, intermediate and/or near without having to resort to using glasses. Monovision gives the presbyopic patient more flexibility with their vision, and allows near vision tasks such as seeing the dashboard of your car, computer screens, menus, price tags, etcetera, without having to reach for a pair of reading glasses. Some people are not able to tolerate monovision for a variety of reasons. The most common is that they feel that while the distance and near vision are okay, neither is crisp enough for their satisfaction since they are using only one eye for each task. Other patients feel "out of balance," nauseated, or as if they have lost their depth perception (for example, the ability to see where one step ends and the next begins in a set of stairs). If carefully measured, all monovision patients will have some loss of depth perception, but those who tolerate it do not notice this.

Due to the downsides to monovision, not every patient will tolerate it. Women, patients with easy-going personalities, and patients with non-technical jobs tend to tolerate monovision better than men, patients who are very detail-oriented, and those with very technical jobs (like engineers). Here are some generalizations: for those over forty years of age, about 25% of my male patients and about 70% of my female patients are successful monovision patients. Why are females more tolerant? We do not know for sure, but perhaps their brains are more flexible. Patients who have vertigo or have one eye that does not see as well as the other eye with glasses on (a condition known in medical terms as amblyopia, or in lay terms "lazy eye"—not to be confused with crossed eyes) are typically not good candidates for monovision. Patients who have successfully worn monovision in contact lenses are excellent candidates for monovision after surgical vision correction.

Should you opt for monovision? The only way to answer this question is to demonstrate it to you. If you are age forty or over, we will help you answer that question as part of the complete pre-operative exam. At this exam, we will demonstrate monovision for you with a pair of trial glasses and give you the opportunity to walk around the office and look at distance, intermediate (computer), and near (reading) targets. Those who adapt to monovision tend to do so very quickly and only require a few minutes to adjust.

Understand that monovision is better tolerated after surgery or with contact lenses than with the trial glasses you might experiment with in the doctor's office, since the glasses can slightly distort vision and magnify the difference between the far and near eye. Those who do well with the trial glasses (i.e., are happy with their distance and near vision) are excellent candidates for monovision. For those patients who are still not sure or wish to spend more time with monovision, we can dispense trial contact lenses at no additional charge for you to test monovision at home and at work. For those of you who have never worn contacts, we are happy to put the contacts in and remove them for you.

While some people may have slight irritation with contacts, we encourage patients to try to pay attention to the vision and ignore the irritation with the contacts while they are in. Also understand that if we perform your surgery as monovision, and you cannot adapt (which happens less than 3% of the time because of the extensive pre-operative testing), we can easily go back and take away the monovision with laser vision correction retreatment. Since it is easier to create monovision at the time of the original surgery than afterwards, we do our best upfront (with trial glasses and/or trial contacts) to make sure that you are a good candidate for monovision.

The amount of monovision given in the reading eye depends on your age and your visual needs. Nearly all of your reading vision will be lost by age fifty to fifty-five. Full monovision is usually created for patients over age fifty. Partial monovision (where the near eye is given some reading, but not full reading to maintain some distance) is frequently employed in younger patients. Partial monovision patients may lose some reading vision with age, but the reading eye will always have some near benefit. As you age, additional reading power can be added to the near eye with laser vision correction. Please keep in mind the more reading power one gets in an eye, the poorer the distance.

Monovision creates flexible, blended vision for both distance and near but does not absolutely guarantee that you will never need glasses for any activities. While many monovision patients never wear glasses, some people find they need a thin pair of night driving glasses that improve distance vision in the near eye for long-distance driving or night-driving in unfamiliar areas. Other patients (particularly partial monovision patients) wear part-time reading glasses that improve the close-up vision in the distance eye for small print, low light situations, and when they do prolonged reading. Other patients who have full monovision may develop an intermediate blur area that requires part-time computer glasses as they age, depending on font size and computer working distance.

Let me describe my own personal experience with monovision. In January 1997, I underwent LASIK in both eyes for distance and ended up with perfect 20/20 vision that has remained stable. One week after my forty-fifth birthday, I noticed that I could no longer comfortably read the newspaper, even though my distance vision was great. I very reluctantly went to the drugstore to get the lowest strength reading glasses. My then-nine-year-old daughter Abigail asked me why I needed glasses since I was a LASIK surgeon. "Honey," I said embarrassedly, "I guess Daddy's eyes are getting old."

My next step was to give trial monovision in trial glasses and contact lenses a shot. Despite being a male ophthalmologist, I liked the improved near vision and did not mind the slight decrease in distance. I went back to my original surgeon twelve years later and had a LASIK enhancement to set my right eye for partial monovision. It was wonderful to personally re-experience exactly what my patients experience every day. By the day after surgery, my near vision was great with only mild decreased distance that I noticed only when I covered my distance eye. Over the weeks after surgery, my brain easily adapted to the new situation. Hooray! I was free of glasses again!

I am now a few years past the surgery for partial monovision (only 0.50 D) and, while I can read, see the computer, and my iPhone without glasses, I find that a low-power pair of drugstore readers improves my close vision, especially for low-light situations, small or low-contrast print, or extended reading. (In fact, patients will likely see me wearing drugstore readers when I am reviewing charts in the dimly lit exam rooms.) While I could have opted for more monovision correction initially to completely eliminate the need for any help with close vision, I did not like the drop in distance vision that I experienced in the trial frame for full monovision. I am quite pleased with the balance that I currently have with the partial monovision.

For patients who do not tolerate monovision, but want to maintain good reading and computer vision after surgery, another option (that can be demonstrated with glasses or contacts) is called a bilateral under correction, where both eyes are set symmetrically for close vision. This situation is ideal for some patients who do a lot of near tasks such as reading/computer use at work but do not need detailed far distance vision without glasses (i.e., pharmacists, manicurists, computer programmers). This allows people to function at work and at home with good close vision and adequate distance vision out to ten to fifteen feet (depending on your preference—the better the near, the poorer the distance). Distance glasses will be required in this situation for activities like driving, sporting events, movies, and so forth.

The last option for maintaining reading vision after vision surgery is with a lens exchange surgery featuring a presbyopic IOL. This surgery is usually reserved for patients over forty-five to fifty that may have early cataracts, but it can also be done in patients who have no cataracts. The natural lens of the eye, which becomes less flexible as you age, is replaced with a new lens which flexes (accommodates) to enhance near vision (Nanoflex, Softec HD, or Crystalens) or a lens that splits light (multi-focal) to see distance and near at the same time (Restore or Tecnis).

Near-vision enhanced lenses like Nanoflex, Softec HD, or the Crystalens allow for excellent distance and intermediate vision, as well as a little bit of near vision in some patients. These lenses are either soft and flexible or have hinges, which we think allows them to move forward when the ciliary muscle in the eye contracts to see better near, and then move backwards for distance vision when the ciliary muscle relaxes, much like the lens of a younger patient. Unlike monovision, both eyes are set the same, and flex equally during the near effort. These lenses are very effective at giving good distance and intermediate vision without glasses following surgery. However, in many patients with these near-enhanced IOLs, part-time reading glasses for fine print and in low light conditions will almost always be necessary, unless partial monovision is employed.

The multifocal lenses Restor and Tecnis are more effective at eliminating the need for reading glasses in most situations. However, because these lenses split light into distance and near components, some patients will have unwanted side effects like glare and halo in low lights or at night. For this reason, these lenses are not implanted in patients who spend a fair amount of time in low-light conditions, or do a significant amount of night driving like truck drivers or policeman who work night shift. In addition, because these multi-focal lenses reduce contrast sensitivity, we do not use them for patients with any ocular condition that can result in reduced contrast, such as previous RK, macular degeneration, or severe dry eyes.

15

Common Misconceptions about Vision Correction Surgery

Eyes are the windows to the soul. They are the magical portals that make possible our perhaps most important sense: sight. Our eyes not only see, they smile. They sparkle. They dance.

It's no wonder, then, that we are so protective of our eyes, and tend to be skeptical of something as understandably frightening as surgery on them.

However, the many misconceptions that have sprung up around vision correction surgery are just that: misconceptions.

To put the minds of prospective patients at ease, I think it's important to explore some of the most common misapprehensions in detail.

Vision correction surgery is not stable

Every surgery I perform, whether lens- or laser-based, involves a permanent change in the vision and is typically stable long-term. After the early to mid-twenties, a patient's prescription remains relatively stable, with the exception of the expected loss of accommodation that occurs in one's forties (which does not change the distance prescription). With laser vision correction (LASIK and PRK), some patients can get some drift in effect towards the original prescription due to healing of the surface cells (epithelium) into areas where tissue has been removed from the cornea with the laser, particularly with farsighted and high nearsighted and high astigmatism treatments. This drift is usually small and typically never so much that it takes the patient back to where he or she started. Regardless, this circumstance is easily corrected with additional laser vision correction.

Lens treatments are even more stable. After Vista Vision ICL, the only reason someone's distance prescription might change is if they develop a cataract, which is a normal part of aging. In this case, cataract surgery with IOL is performed to restore the vision. As previously discussed, lens exchange (cataract surgery with an IOL) is the ultimate vision correction procedure. Anyone who lives to be old enough will eventually need this procedure—which is certainly preferable to the alternative of not living to be old enough! Once the natural lens has been removed and replaced with an IOL, the vision will remain stable.

My prescription is not stable

While I will not perform surgery on patient whose prescription is not stable, many patients come to me with the mistaken belief that their prescription isn't stable. Stability is defined as one diopter or less of change in the prescription over the previous year. This is exceptionally unusual in patients older than their teens or early twenties. Because the accuracy of testing refractive error (glasses prescription) is not perfect, with some variability from visit to visit, you may have some minor changes from year to year that are of no significance. In some circumstances, patients are told that "they need new glasses" even though there has been only a minor change that will not really make a difference for them. Such minor changes do not represent instability that would prevent you from having surgery.

The best way to determine your own stability is to check your vision with your current glasses or contacts; if you are unstable and have had a significant change, you would not be able to function visually with your current prescription. Regardless, we will carefully check your stability by reviewing the power in the glasses you bring with you, as well as reviewing any information we can obtain about old prescriptions. If you have an optometrist who you have seen more than once who has referred you, he/she would have already checked the stability of your vision before making the referral.

I am too young to have vision correction surgery

"You're never too young to fall in love," goes an old saying. When it comes to vision correction surgery, however, there is a standard I adhere to. In normal circumstances, I will perform vision correction surgery in patients as young as age seventeen, as long as the glasses/contact prescription is stable (see above). In the FDA studies for all vision correction technologies, patients were required to be twenty-one years of age or older to eliminate any question of stability that might affect the outcomes, meaning that the surgeries are "labeled" for patients twenty-one and up. As discussed previously, surgery on patients under twenty-one is therefore considered "off-label." However, I have routinely and successfully corrected many patients under twenty-one with LASIK, PRK, and Vista Vision ICL. I am more likely to perform surgery on younger patients when the patient is highly motivated or there is a compelling reason to perform surgery; for instance, a high school football quarterback who is contact lens-intolerant and can't wear glasses under his helmet. With any patient under twenty-five, I will advise them that they have a higher risk of needing additional treatment (as compared to a patient over this age) down the road if their prescription changes slightly as their eye develops. However, the rate of late retreatment in younger patients is still quite low. If LASIK technology were available when I was seventeen, I would have gladly undergone surgery to eliminate the need for glasses throughout my twenties despite the slightly higher risk of needing additional treatment later in life.

I am too old to have vision correction surgery

Just like the dog that isn't too old to learn a new trick or two, no one is too old for vision correction surgery. The oldest patient I have done LASIK/PRK on is eighty-eight; the oldest I have perfomed ICL on is sixty-six; and the oldest I have performed lensectomy/IOL on is—are you ready for this?—103. In my practice, more mature patients are just as happy after surgery as my younger patients! The main issue affecting the vision correction candidacy of older patients is whether or not they have cataracts. I closely screen for cataracts in anyone age forty-five or older. If I determine that you have any level of cataract, then the procedure that I would recommend for you would be lensectomy (cataract surgery) with an IOL to correct your vision. The beauty of being diagnosed with a cataract is that your non-HMO medical insurance will help pay for the vision correction surgery and make the price of one of the newer premium IOLs more in line with the costs of LASIK.

My prescription is too low to have surgery

This is another common misnomer. Any patient with any prescription who is dependent on glasses or contacts to see is a candidate for surgery. Just because the prescription is low does not eliminate you as a candidate. Only you can be the judge; if you are happy with your vision without glasses or contacts, there is no need for surgery. In my own personal case, I had a very low prescription in my right eye before my LASIK (-1.00 diopters). Despite this low prescription, I constantly wore glasses or contacts to improve my vision. My decision to have LASIK was one of the wisest choices I have ever made in my life.

My prescription is too high to have surgery

With modern technology, virtually any prescription can be corrected, including extremely high prescriptions. The average patient (meaning near-sighted) I perform LASIK on is 3.00 diopters. For high prescriptions, lens surgery (ICL or IOL) is a much better alternative than LASIK/PRK. I recently performed ICL surgery followed three months later by PRK on a patient from Turkey who had a prescription of -23.00 diopters. Every surgeon that she saw in her native country told her that there was nothing that could be done for her vision other than contact lenses, which constantly moved and blurred because of her unusually steep corneas. After her surgery, she saw better in each eye than she ever had with glasses or contacts! Another example: I recently performed a successful vision correction surgery on a woman who was -27.00 diopters in her only eye, which also had a cataract! Because of her huge prescription, she needed a minus (reverse) power IOL with implantation of an ICL at the same surgery because she needed a minus power IOL higher than what is manufactured by any company. Proof positive that no prescription is too high for current lens technology.

Astigmatism cannot be corrected

This is simply not true. Virtually any level of astigmatism can safely and effectively be corrected with multiple vision correction technologies including LASIK, PRK, Vista Vision ICL with limbal relaxing incisions, and toric IOLs. Astigmatic LASIK is highly successful and has been FDA approved for over a decade. While highly successful, the necessity of correcting astigmatism at the time of LASIK does slightly increase the risk of enhancement surgery (retreatment) and the risk of night glare/halo compared to nearsighted LASIK. Compared to toric (astigmatic-treating) soft lenses, which often rotate and blur, most patients prefer the vision they get after vision correction surgery to their toric contacts.

I cannot have surgery because I am nursing

While nursing mothers were excluded from LASIK and ICL FDA trials because of the theoretical risk of change in prescription after hormones change when nursing is discontinued, I have performed countless vision correction procedures on nursing mothers with stable results. While these treatments are "off-label," I have never seen significant refractive changes when the mother has stopped nursing. While I will not do surgery on pregnant women—both because of the risk of vision changes related to changes in blood sugar associated with pregnancy, and because of the risk to the fetus related to relaxing medication at the time of surgery—the same thing does not hold true for nursing mothers. In many circumstances, I have successfully treated mothers who are looking to grow a large family; these women typically serially nurse and then get pregnant, and would essentially never have the opportunity to correct their vision until much later in life if FDA labeling was followed. If a sedative like Valium or Xanax is taken, it is important that the mother store milk prior to the procedure for use after the procedure, as these medications are secreted in the breast milk for up to forty-eight hours.

83

I should wait for surgery because technology is always changing

In our technology-crazed culture, where today's "it" product every-body has to have is tomorrow's "boat anchor," it is sometimes prudent to wait and see if that gadget you're salivating over has staying power. However, this does not really apply to vision correction surgeries. The current technologies we have for vision correction procedures are excellent, and are not likely to change significantly over the next five to ten years (see the last chapter). Waiting for surgery because of new technology is much like saying you will wait to buy a computer because software and hardware is constantly evolving. While this is certainly true, current computer technology works well and future changes should not stop you from purchasing a computer.

As a member of the editorial board of our refractive surgery scientific journal, and by looking to foreign countries that have access to technologies long before they become FDA approved, I can look into the future of our field. While there may be some minor changes in the laser and lens delivery systems and microkeratomes, LASIK and ICL have been very safe and effective treatments since they were developed in the mid-1990s and will not likely change significantly for the average patient. The successful LASIK procedure I had on my own eyes in 1997 is only minimally different from the LASIK procedure that is offered today, some fifteen years later. If there is a technology that will be available in the future that will make a significant difference to a patient, I will certainly make the recommendation to wait for that technology—but this represents less than 1% of the patients I encounter, typically those who have had issues with previous eye surgery or have the disease keratoconus.

I can't have surgery because I have a lazy eye

This is a common misconception from two standpoints. First of all, most people think that a "lazy eye" is an eye that crosses. The true definition of lazy eye or amblyopia is an eye that looks normal but cannot see 20/20 even with glasses. Lazy eye is a brain phenomenon where the eye cannot be corrected to 20/20, rather than a wandering eye (technically termed a "strabismus" or muscle imbalance). I routinely treat patients with strabismus and with lazy eye. If the strabismus is corrected when glasses or contacts are worn—that is, farsighted patients whose eyes turn inward unless they are wearing glasses or contacts—then the strabismus will also be corrected with vision correction surgery. If the eye still crosses when glasses or contacts are worn, then the strabismus will persist after surgery. I will recommend to some patients with this situation to consider eye muscle surgery prior to vision correction surgery.

The second misconception with lazy eye (amblyopia) is that refractive surgery cannot be performed. I can and do routinely perform vision correction surgery on lazy eyes. The main issue with this situation is that I can never get the vision better after vision correction surgery than it was with the best pair of glasses or contacts. That is to say, if the patient was only correctable to 20/40, a patient could only expect a 20/40 outcome after LASIK or other procedure in that eye. The other issue is that while risks are very low, the patient with lazy eye is taking a risk on the eye with good corrected vision if they have both eyes corrected. If the lazy eye were so dense that the patient could not function if the lazy eye were their only eye, I would usually recommend against vision correction surgery except in unusual circumstances where the patient has a compelling reason to proceed with surgery. I once had a patient who had very dense lazy eye in one eye (which was legally blind, even with glasses) and a high nearsighted prescription in the fellow eye. He was an avid skier and swimmer who reluctantly had to give up these activities because he was contact lens-intolerant. Aware of his desire to return to these activities, I was willing to perform surgery on him with appropriate informed consent, and he was soon zooming down the slopes and zipping across the pool after successful surgery.

I can't have surgery because I have had previous eye surgery

I humbly beg to differ! I routinely perform surgery on patients who have previous eye surgery including LASIK, PRK, RK, cataract surgery, corneal transplants, strabismus surgery, and retinal detachment surgery. I will explore these unique circumstances in the next chapter.

16

Vision Correction Surgery After Previous Eye Surgery

Surgery after LASIK/PRK

With over seven million corneal refractive procedures having been performed in the United States, the most common circumstance I encounter in patients with previous eye surgery who come in for consultation is when they have had previous LASIK or PRK. Fortunately, this is typically a straightforward circumstance, unless the patient has irregularity of the cornea from a previous treatment. In this circumstance, I recommend that the patient wait for topography-guided laser technology to perform the procedure (see the next chapter). The more common situation is where the vision is easily treated with currently available technology. If the LASIK is less than three to four years old and there is adequate corneal thickness, I will lift the previous flap and apply additional laser treatment. If the patient has had PRK, or the LASIK flap is more than three to four years old, I will perform surface laser treatment (PRK or LASEK, which is PRK with alcohol applied at the time of surgery to loosen the surface cells). As described earlier, the main downside of surface treatment is slow vision recovery, but it is quite effective at restoring good vision.

Surgery after Radial Keratotomy (RK)

Additional refractive surgery after LASIK is more challenging than other circumstances, but is still extremely effective. Because RK was done routinely from the early 1980s to the mid-1990s and weakens the cornea, many of these patients come in with farsighted prescriptions and early cataracts because they are age fifty and older, making lensectomy/IOL my procedure of choice for the majority of them. In many of these circumstances, insurance will get involved in paying for the procedure.

There are three issues with performing lens surgery in RK patients. The first is the accuracy of the procedure. Because of the previous corneal surgery, the lens calculation used to pick the correct IOL power is much more difficult than if the patient had not had surgery. We employ special tests to help improve the accuracy of the calculation, but there is still a high risk of needing additional treatment with surface PRK. In fact, I tell RK patients undergoing lensectomy/IOL to expect a two-stage operation, with the PRK occurring three months after the lens procedure.

The second issue is that RK patients take longer to heal after lensectomy/IOL surgery because of swelling of the RK incisions that creates flattening of the cornea and induced astigmatism and/or farsightedness, requiring a few months to stabilize.

The last issue with lens surgery in RK patients is the fact that sometimes the previous incisions will open at the time of lens surgery, requiring sutures to close them that can induce astigmatism. While I place the opening into the eye for cataract surgery as far away from the RK incisions as possible, this still sometimes occurs. Fortunately, the sutures are removed in the first few months and any residual astigmatism is very treatable with additional PRK.

In younger RK patients who do not have a high farsighted prescription or early cataracts, I use PRK as my primary treatment. LASIK has been used in the past, but there is a very high risk of the previous incisions opening, which can allow cells to grow from the surface under the flap (epithelial ingrowth). Significant epithelial ingrowth can create flap melts, induced astigmatism, and blurry vision, requiring additional surgery. Performing PRK on previous RK patients avoids this issue. While PRK on an RK eye is slightly less accurate than on a virgin cornea, resulting in a higher enhancement rate for these eyes, PRK is safe and highly effective.

Surgery after cataract/IOL

Many patients will end up with the need for glasses or contacts after cataract surgery, particularly if the surgeon does not offer premium IOLs. Further surgery to correct any residual prescription is relatively straightforward, and the type of surgery is dependent upon the size of the residual prescription. For most nearsighted, farsighted, and astigmatic prescriptions, laser vision correction with LASIK or PRK may be performed, assuming that there has been at least a three-month period since the cataract surgery has been performed in order to allow the incision to heal. Prior to performing LASIK/PRK, it is also important to make sure that any clouding of the capsule that holds the IOL in place (called a posterior capsular opacity, which is very common after cataract surgery and easily cleared with a two-minute, in-office procedure called a YAG capsulotomy) is cleared. The choice as to whether LASIK and PRK is performed is identical to the decision made for patients who have never had surgery—i.e., those with thin or asymmetrically shaped corneas or a history of significant dry eye are advised to have PRK instead of LASIK. The outcomes in LASIK/PRK for patients who have cataract surgery are excellent and comparable to patients who have never had any surgery performed on their eyes.

In the unusual circumstance where a patient has an extremely large prescription after cataract surgery, I typically perform lens exchange or lens piggyback. Lens exchange involves removing the old IOL and replacing it with a new lens with the proper power. This is most easily accomplished in the first two to four weeks after the original surgery, because beyond this point, the lens usually seals into the capsular bag (the membrane that holds the IOL in place) and is more difficult to remove. In these circumstances, a second (or piggyback) lens is placed on top of the old lens. Both procedures are typically performed under eye drop anesthesia and take five to ten minutes, with good outcome.

Surgery after corneal transplantation

Typically after corneal transplantation, the patient is left with a large amount of astigmatism as well as nearsightedness or farsightedness, requiring a contact lens to see well. In these circumstances, as long as the patient is correctable with glasses (that is, does not have too much irregularity of the new cornea due to healing issues), laser vision correction is a good option. I typically perform PRK in these circumstances because of the higher risk of an irregular flap or epithelial ingrowth when creating a LASIK flap over a previous transplant. While many patients do well with PRK over a transplant, the risk of needing a secondary (enhancement) treatment is higher with a transplant than in a virgin cornea.

Surgery after strabismus surgery

Vision correction surgery after strabismus (eye muscle) surgery is no different in terms of risks or outcomes than surgery performed on a virgin eye. The main issue is to make sure that ocular alignment with the strabismus surgery is normalized before proceeding with the vision correction surgery.

Surgery after retinal detachment surgery

The three basic ways of surgically treating a retinal detachment are pneumatic retinopexy (placing air into the eye followed by laser treatment of the retinal break), scleral buckling (placing a plastic buckle around the outside of the eye), and vitrectomy (surgical removal of the vitreous jelly of the eye and lasering the retinal break). Lens- and laser-based vision correction surgery after pneumatic retinopexy is no different than surgery in a virgin eye both in terms of risk or outcome.

A scleral buckle frequently causes lengthening of the entire eye due to mid-eye pressure with the buckle, resulting in nearsightedness. IOL/ICL surgery after a scleral buckle is no different than in a virgin eye. However, LASIK may become more difficult because the buckle can interfere with the achievement of suction with the microkeratome to create the flap. In some circumstances, the keratome will not attach to the eye, and LASIK is not possible, requiring PRK or ICL instead of LASIK.

Lastly, eyes which have had a vitrectomy respond to LASIK/PRK identically as virgin eyes, but are typically at much higher risk of having a cataract after the vitrectomy, making lensectomy/IOL a much more common procedure in these eyes. Lens surgery is slightly more difficult in these patients because the natural lens can move more than usual due to a lack of the vitreous jelly, which stabilizes the lens during surgery.

17

What about Future Technology?

"The future cannot be predicted, but futures can be invented."
—*Dennis Gabor,* Inventing the Future *(1964)*

Today, we take for granted enjoying many of the technological advancements in medicine, engineering, and electronics that popular culture phenomena like TV's *Star Trek* first predicted some forty years ago. Similarly, since I did my refractive surgery fellowship in 1993, refractive surgery has been developing at warp speed and is now a completely different field than back in those early years. In 1993, the main refractive procedure was radial keratotomy (radial incisions in the cornea to weaken it to treat nearsightedness). RK has subsequently been abandoned because 30 to 50% of patients developed progressive flattening of the eye, causing hyperopia or farsightedness (progressive hyperopic shift). I am now fixing the vision in many of these patients with PRK or lensectomy/IOL. When I performed my first PRK in 1993, the excimer laser was still in its infancy (it had first been used on sighted eyes in 1987, and the first LASIK performed in 1991) and was undergoing FDA trials. In fact, at Phillips Eye Institute where I trained, we had the largest series of laser patients in the United States during those trials. The field of refractive surgery at that time was not even a sub-specialty, and no one practiced refractive surgery full-time.

In 1995, the excimer laser was first approved for use with PRK. A short time later, surgeons were using the keratome to create a flap in an off-label procedure called LASIK, which was not approved by the FDA until 1999. By 1999, at least ten companies had been formed to provide LASIK to the public (many of which subsequently went bankrupt) and LASIK became well known, with references in the news media, television, and movies. Many surgeons became full-time refractive surgeons, making refractive surgery a sub-specialty of ophthalmology.

By 2005, the ICL was approved for the treatment of patients outside the range of LASIK. In 2009, LASIK volumes were down 40-50%, while ICL volumes were up 25%. Despite this fact, most surgeons still have not accepted ICL as a mainstream alternative to LASIK. In my practice this is one of the things that I am working to change. This is because ICL is a more technically demanding surgery, and most surgeons are now just taking the training course (many of them in my Los Angeles office).

Where do I see the field of refractive surgery going in the future? I think that the ICL procedure will replace LASIK as the procedure of choice at all ranges of approval (moderate nearsightedness [-3] and above) because of the advantages discussed previously. Given that 50% of patients who undergo vision surgery are low myopes (under -3D) LASIK and PRK will still be very commonly performed on these patients. Because we get such great results with the current lasers and keratomes at these levels, LASIK will not change much in the foreseeable future. Perhaps small modifications in the lasers and keratomes will make the procedure a little safer and a little more accurate, but it will be hard to improve upon what is currently available.

One laser technology that is likely to be widely adopted in the near future is one called topography-guided LASIK, of which I was one of the lead investigators in the United States; hopefully we will see approval by the FDA at some point in the near future. Current "wavefront-guided" lasers utilize only 200 data points in an attempt to improve vision quality and lessen night vision symptoms after LASIK by minimizing induction of HOAs and reducing HOAs. Topo-guided LASIK utilizes 7000 data points to measure and treat the HOAs—much higher fidelity than currently available lasers. As a result, in our FDA study of this technology, over half of the eyes achieved "super-vision" (vision better than 20/20) and we were able to reduce the 24% of patients who complained of night glare/halo with glasses/contacts to 0% after the LASIK. Importantly, this was actually the first time in the history of LASIK where we were consistently improving, rather than diminishing, night vision. This technology is also very useful for correcting vision in patients who have ended up with irregular treatments or worsened night vision. While this is better technology for certain patients with irregular corneas, for the average patient, it does not necessarily give a better outcome than currently available lasers.

The other changes in technology that I see in the future have to do with use of IOLs, especially with regard to correcting presbyopia. Over the past few years, use of IOLs (refractive lensectomy) has increased dramatically in our field because of the superior quality of vision compared to LASIK, the permanence of the procedure (you will never significantly change prescription or develop a cataract), and the emergence of presbyopic-treating IOLs. I predict that current-generation multi-focal IOLs will be used less often because they create artificial optics with the potential for decreased contrast sensitivity and poor night vision and a single point of near focus. As they improve, accommodating (near-enhancing) IOLs will become the technology of the future and will be offered to every patient over age forty-eight to fifty to correct their vision, regardless of prescription.

Eventually (though not in our lifetime) these accommodating IOLs or lens replacement materials will closely simulate the eye of a twenty-year-old, allowing 100% of the population to consider these lenses when they become presbyopic. While the currently available near-enhancing lenses (I prefer the Nanoflex and Softec HD over the FDA-labeled Crystalens) are very good, these lenses have the main downside of not accommodating enough, requiring reading glasses some or all of the time. There are newer generations of accommodating IOLs in the pipeline, but their clinical utility remains to be seen. In my opinion, the most promising is the Tetraflex IOL by Lenstec. This IOL is easier to for the surgeon to insert and has a larger optic surface, (which may reduce the risks of night glare) than the currently FDA-labeled Crystalens.

You may wonder: What does the future hold for Dr. Paul Dougherty? Well, one thing for certain will never change: I love interacting with patients as a refractive surgeon. I love the positive life change that I make for humans every day with current technologies. I will continue to do surgery, at least part-time, until I am no longer physically able. I currently develop technologies with industry leaders (topo-guided LASIK, ICL, and Tetraflex) and would love to continue and expand these relationships. As part of the development process, I conduct clinical research and publish my findings in peer-reviewed journals, as well as serving on their editorial boards in many cases. I will continue this and would like to expand my role as a researcher, author, and lecturer.

I am currently in the process of developing the first-of-its-kind ICL/IOL-focused refractive surgery center in the United States. After proof of concept in the Los Angeles market, I plan on expanding these centers around the country. I have a passion for teaching, and have taught my techniques to thousands of surgeons around the globe (Asia, Europe, Middle East, Australia, and South America) and hope to continue this outreach. In developing ICL/IOL surgery centers, I will be able to pursue my passion for teaching by developing new surgical talent for each new center by personally teaching young surgeons my techniques and philosophies.

Lastly, my biggest pleasure in life is to give my gift of vision correction to those who cannot afford it. I want to help eliminate every treatable cause of blindness in this world—namely refractive error and cataracts. I am developing my national chain of ICL/IOL refractive surgery centers as the economic engine to fund my passion. World Vision Project (discussed in depth in the next chapter) is underway now, starting to make my vision a reality. As someone who believes in a higher being and believes that I am part of this higher being, I will thus be achieving my highest self-actualization through my service.

18

My Vision for the
Future/Philanthropy

My Vision is Global Vision. My profession of vision correction surgery has afforded me many extraordinary experiences and introduced me to many wonderful patients. Because of this, I want to give something of lasting value back to the world.

In 2010, I formed an international charitable organization called World Vision Project. It is currently being incorporated as a U.S. 501c3 non-profit. According to the World Health Organization, the leading cause of avoidable global blindness is cataracts. The centerpiece of World Vision Project is surgical vision correction (primarily cataract surgery) and other medical services for often indigent and incredibly deserving patients, notably in association with local physicians and hospital staff who can help to improve and sustain higher quality care in their communities.

In the past, I have worked with many other charitable organizations to achieve my philanthropic goals. Over the past five years, I have worked with the Ventura County Community College District to give free LASIK to one deserving, underprivileged student at each of the three Ventura County community colleges: Ventura, Moorpark, and Oxnard. Every year, students from each college submit applications outlining why they are deserving of this award.

Perhaps my most touching moment in this program came in 2003 when a young student from Oxnard was awarded LASIK. He was one of eleven children in a family whose father earned $12,000 a year as a gardener. This student was the first in his family to ever attend college, and while he was a serious scholar, his passion in life was unquestionably baseball. He had given up playing the game when he developed nearsightedness, requiring glasses. Because of his family's financial situation, he could not risk playing the game and breaking his glasses. I wish you could have seen the tears in the eyes of the student and his father after the procedure, which went flawlessly. It still gives me goose bumps.

As part of World Vision Project, we also routinely gift LASIK surgery during armed forces weekend to severely wounded veterans from the Wounded Warrior Transition Facility in Ft. Hood, Texas, in association with Herosnightout.org and the Motorcycle Charity Foundation.

In 2008, I worked with Bausch and Lomb, Inc., which organized an innovative charitable project known as "Changing 100 Lives in 100 Minutes" in celebration of the one hundred thousandth Crystalens accommodating intraocular lens (IOL) implant. B&L donated one hundred pairs of the lenses to low-income people across the United States, and an equal number of ophthalmologists performed implantation surgeries from coast to coast over the course of an hour and forty minutes, at no charge. The event took place on April 9. For more information, see this link:

www.bausch.com.ar/en_US/corporate/corpcomm/news/
crystalens_100people100minutes.aspx

As one of the surgeons in the project, I had the opportunity to operate on both eyes of a patient in her early fifties who worked as a housekeeper. She had farsightedness and cataracts in both eyes, and she had never been able to afford to see an eye doctor or to get glasses for her farsightedness. When I first saw her, she was wearing a pair of glasses borrowed from a friend that were not even the correct prescription. Tragically, she told me she had never seen clearly as an adult. I performed cataract surgery with Crystalens implants on both eyes on that fateful April day, allowing her to see clearly distance and near without glasses for the first time in her adult life. What a positive, life-changing experience for patient and doctor.

My staff and I also work with Mission Cataract USA (www.missioncataractusa .org) whose goal is to eliminate blindness in the United States from cataracts (clouding of the natural lens of the eye). In concert with Mission Cataract USA and Staar Surgical, Inc, we routinely provide free eye surgery for those who do not have the ability to pay. One day each quarter is designated for such patients at my Advanced Sight Surgery Center in Los Angeles.

Every year since 2008, on Thanksgiving Day, Dougherty Laser Vision teams with The Westside Thanksgiving Day Dinner Committee to provide free eye care to the homeless at the Santa Monica Civic Arts Auditorium. This annual event provides food, clothing, blankets, haircuts, make-up, and medical care (including flu shots) for the homeless. At the event, my colleagues and I perform eye exams and give away eye drops for patients with dry eyes, allergies, and glaucoma. Eyeglasses donated from LASIK patients at Dougherty Laser Vision are given to patients with matching prescriptions.

At this event in 2009, I met a homeless man in his forties with a very high prescription in his glasses who attributed his homelessness to his lifetime poor vision. I was lucky enough to be able to gift him Vista Vision ICL surgery in both of his eyes, and he is now seeing almost 20/20 without his glasses. This ability that I was given to change lives in a positive way through restorative vision surgery never fails to warm my heart and has put my life's work into sharp focus.

In September of 2010, as part of World Vision Project, my staff and I worked in concert with UNRWA (The United Nations Relief and Works Organization) and Project-Peace on Earth to gift forty cataract surgeries to visually impaired Palestinian refugees in the West Bank city of Hebron. My staff and I were fortunate enough to work with the staff and facilities of St. John Eye Hospital in Jerusalem, and we could not have achieved all that we did without the generous support of the Bank of Palestine and a long list of local partners.

The trip was truly an eye-opening experience for my staff and me as we witnessed firsthand what is really happening on the ground in the region; especially enlightening were the shared experiences of many different people with respect to future peace in the Middle East. With great anticipation we look forward to our future World Vision Project trips to gift surgical vision correction. My most heartfelt thanks goes out to everyone—patients, peers, sponsors, and donors—who enable me to give something back to deserving people around the globe.

My goal for World Vision Project is to grow it into the premier philanthropic eye surgery institution in the world, helping people with poor vision—who cannot afford to pay for eye surgery—to realize the life-altering benefits of modern cataract and refractive surgery, both in the United States and around the world.

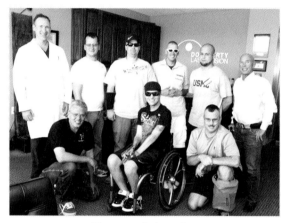

The wounded warriors

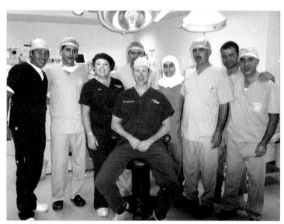

With my U.S. and Palestinian surgical team,
Hebron, West Bank. September 2010

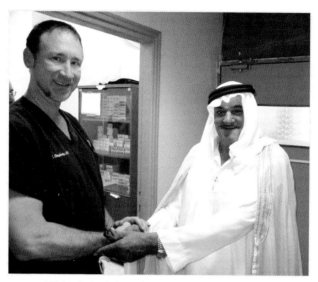

With a Palestinian tribal leader before his surgery

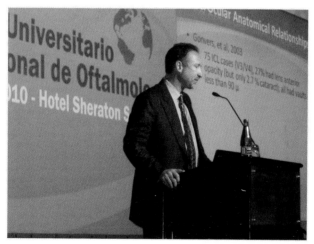

Lecturing to the Chilean Ophthalmological Society,
Santiago, Chile. July 2010

Afterword

A number of years ago, I had the pleasure of meeting spiritual teachers David and Margaret Hiller and gifting LASIK to David. As someone who believes from a spiritual standpoint that there are no coincidences in this life and that everything happens exactly the way it should, I was quite honored and humbled by the section that David added to his book about his experience with vision correction surgery. What follows is an excerpt from his book, *Dare to Dream*.

As We Perceive, So Shall We Receive

by David Hiller

I have worn glasses since I was six years old in the first grade. Most of us who have worn glasses remember the kidding we got from some of the children at school and how that made us feel. One of the things I heard a lot was, "David, you sure look funny with four eyes!" Some of us learned how to hide behind our glasses because we were not being seen for who we truly were, and it felt like we needed to protect ourselves from the world. We then began to see ourselves through other people's eyes.

To a certain extent, that was the case for me, and I became very shy and introverted in the classroom. Interestingly, however, I turned to sports to be more recognized. I was very athletic and never wore my glasses while playing sports. I felt so much better about myself then and received a lot of acceptance and encouragement. This, of course, allowed me to see myself in a whole new light!

This "inner sight" also helped me excel at sports even though I had difficulty actually seeing—either the ball or the other players—without my glasses! I developed a kind of inner instinct to move or react at just the right time to succeed at what I was doing. By the time I graduated from college that inner instinct was highly developed. It helped me to be much more extroverted even though I was still wearing glasses and sometimes hiding behind them when I felt uncomfortable in another's presence.

I dreamed that one day a miracle would happen and I would no longer need to wear glasses, that I would have 20/20 vision—perfect eyesight. I knew that this was possible if I continued to develop my inner vision, improve my view of myself, and trust that others could see me more truthfully (as I revealed myself to them more truthfully) whether I wore glasses or not. I began to dream a holier dream, seeing with 20/20 vision both from the inner as well as the outer! I believed that this was possible.

Well, guess what! In October of 2001, about six weeks after the 9/11 tragedy, we were presenting a Sunday service at a church in Ventura, California. I had just finished talking about a powerful healing and forgiveness process I had experienced at a workshop on letting go of old wounds, when a man walked up to me, shook my hand, and told me he felt really inspired by what I said. I held his hand for a minute, looked into his eyes, and felt genuinely acknowledged. I was delighted that my words had touched him.

He then said, "My name is Dr. Paul Dougherty. I'm a laser eye surgeon and medical director of Dougherty Laser Vision in Camarillo, California, and I feel truly inspired to give you a gift! I noticed that you were wearing glasses during your talk and figured you have probably worn them for a long time. Is that true?"

"Yes," I answered, "since I was six years old."

Then I noticed the twinkle in his eyes as he said, "I would like to give you the gift of laser eye surgery so you can have 20/20 vision."

Well, I was stunned and couldn't speak for a couple of seconds! All kinds of thoughts swirled around in my head. Finally, I regained my composure enough to answer a resounding, "Yes, thank you so much, you're an answer to my prayer! I've been dreaming about this for a long time." God sent me an Earth angel to answer my prayers! Paul asked me to come to his office in a couple of days to determine if I was a good candidate for this procedure and I agreed. I could hardly wait to "see" if this was going to work for me, and when the time came, I felt a tremendous excitement.

I arrived at his office and was greeted by very warm and friendly people who made me feel right at home. Everyone was very attentive, which gave me a real sense of security. After all, these were my eyes that were going to be operated on, and I was feeling a little nervous, so the tender loving care was most appreciated! Several of the doctor's assistants checked my eyes, and then Paul came in, looked at my eyes, said that I was a perfect candidate for laser surgery, and that I would be seeing 20/20 very soon. Those words were music to my ears! I was so excited I could hardly contain myself! Paul was so confident, I felt absolutely reassured that I was in good hands, and all my nervousness just melted away.

The next day I returned to the clinic to have the laser procedure done. Margaret came with me for support, but little did she know that she would actually be able to witness the surgery. What a gift! After I was prepped for surgery, Paul told me again that everything was going to be fine, that he would talk me through the entire surgery, and tell me how it was going every step of the way. Again, I felt very reassured and comforted and I said, "I'm ready, let's do it."

The laser surgery was amazing to me. I didn't feel any pain, and Paul talked to me the whole time, which was probably about five minutes for each eye. He kept saying really positive things like, "It's going perfectly. You're doing great, Dave. You'll be seeing 20/20 real soon." I never knew surgery could actually be a pleasant experience!

First, the doctor numbed my eyes with eye drops. Then he used a Keratome, an instrument devised to separate the front layer of the cornea from the rest of the eye to create the corneal flap. The flap was then folded over and an Excimer laser was used to reshape the tissue underneath it. This procedure is quite like sculpting a contact lens on the eye. Then the flap was put back into place where it began to heal immediately and naturally without stitches.

Margaret, who was in the next room, was grateful for the opportunity to watch this entire amazing procedure through a large glass window. What a gift to be able to see this miracle of science performed right before her eyes! After the surgery was over, Paul examined my eyes again and said everything looked great. He told me to go back to our motel and lie down, keeping my eyes closed and covered with protective goggles for the next four hours. Then I could open them to a whole new world!

It seemed like those four hours took an eternity but finally the moment of truth arrived! I slowly took the goggles off, said a prayer and opened my eyes. Lo and behold, I could see perfectly for the first time in my life! I was astonished. It was one of the most precious moments of my life. I'll never forget seeing things so clearly—shapes, colors, words—everything was clearer. I started jumping up and down on the bed like a kid in a candy store, looking at myself in the mirror and seeing one happy camper! I started singing some crazy song that I made up on the spot—I do that sometimes—and that always makes Margaret laugh. We held each other in absolute delight. Later that day we went out to get some sunglasses for me. I'd never worn non-prescription sunglasses before that I could actually see through, and this was a real treat. I started reading various road signs and saw words that even Margaret couldn't see, and she has great long-distance vision. We both got a big kick out of that.

A few days later I spent some time reflecting on what a phenomenal gift it was to receive clear outer vision. I believe the gift came to me because I really worked on self-forgiveness for seeing myself through others' eyes, for letting that affect me so much and sometimes closing down. Forgiveness opened my heart to seeing myself through the eyes of love, thus allowing others the freedom to look more deeply into my eyes, right into my heart and soul. After all, the eyes are the mirrors of the soul, the spiritual, holy, eternal aspect of our being!

I want to thank everyone at Dougherty Laser Vision for their kindness and professionalism and a very special "thank you" to Dr. Paul for the exquisite gift he gave me, for being such a great doctor, and even more importantly, for his heart of gold.

News Articles

Vision Correction Surgery Articles about Los Angeles Vision Surgeon Dr. Paul Dougherty

The Journal of Refractive Surgery Appoints Paul Dougherty, M.D. to Editorial Board Highly Prestigious Honor Reserved for World's Foremost Specialists

PR Newswire

Los Angeles

July 14, 2005

Renowned vision correction surgeon Paul J. Dougherty, M.D. has been selected to serve on the editorial board of the Journal of Refractive Surgery. With this highly prestigious honor, Dr. Dougherty joins an elite group of specialists known internationally for their contributions to the field of vision correction.

The Journal of Refractive Surgery is the official peer-reviewed journal of the American Academy of Ophthalmology and the affiliated International Society of Refractive Surgery. Each bimonthly issue serves as a forum for original research, review and evaluation of refractive and corneal surgery procedures. The Journal's editorial board currently includes just 39 surgeons from around the world, 20 of whom are from the U.S.

"I am very honored to be asked to join such an exclusive group of top surgeons," said Dr. Dougherty. "I look forward to joining colleagues from around the world in helping shape the Journal's coverage of the latest clinical advances."

The Journal of Refractive Surgery is not the first peer-reviewed journal to ask Dr. Dougherty to provide peer review. He also currently serves as a reviewer for the American Journal of Ophthalmology and the Journal of Cataract and Refractive Surgery.

Ophthalmologist's Vision Realized in Implantable Contacts

By Deborah Crowe

Los Angeles Business Journal

Los Angeles

April 2007

Dr. Paul Dougherty carefully makes a 3-millimeter slit near the edge of the cornea of Rod Barshook's right eye and slides a rolled-up contact lens between the iris and the eye's own lens. After the lens unrolls itself, he gently tucks the edges under the iris. A few minutes later another contact is implanted in the other eye.

Less than a half hour later, Barshook sits in a reclining chair at Dougherty's Larchmont Village medical offices; his eyes are still a little blurry from the local anesthetic but he is able to read the clock on the opposite wall without the Coke bottle glasses he's worn most of his life.

"I'm pretty excited," he exclaims about the lens, manufactured by Monrovia-based Staar Surgical Co. It's that "wow factor," as well as positive word-of-mouth and the enthusiasm of ophthalmologists like Dougherty, that Staar is counting on as the cornerstones of the marketing plan for its long-awaited, Visian ICL implantable contact lens.

"I knew this lens was the future," said Dougherty, who has been working with the lens since 1999 when he and handful of other surgeons traveled to Mexico to perform implantations as part of their training. "I knew the limitations of Lasik for people with higher levels of myopia. The further you push LASIK, the less accurate it is. We needed an alternative."

It's been slightly more than three months since U.S. regulators finally approved the ICL, which was already available in 41 other countries. Only a fraction of the U.S. surgeons who have received initial training are now certi-fied to implant the device, and even those who can are only now beginning to receive brochures to distribute to patients.

The small Monrovia-based company employs only seven proctors to oversee the five monitored operations that surgeons have to perform before the company will supply them the lens. The company expects to have only 500 of nearly 1,000 eligible surgeons certified by the end of the year. But management believes the rollout is going just fine.

"It sounds like a crazy situation but it's not really," said Chief Executive David Bailey, who followed a similar strategy when introducing Lasik eye surgery in Europe for another company in the mid-1990s. "A slow, steady ramp-up gives you solid outcomes and happy patients from which you can build the marketing. It's worth it to us in the long run to wait."

The Visian ICL is the first implantable lens for the correction of adult nearsightedness that is foldable, and therefore minimally invasive. It requires an incision about half the size of an older, competing lens marketed by Santa Ana-based Advanced Medical Optics Inc. Unlike refractive surgery, the procedure is reversible and significantly less prone to side effects.

"Doctors are the best people to sell the technology and our role is to support that," said Bailey, noting that for the initial rollout, surgeons with large refractive surgery practices have been targeted. "It's a very easy product to market because the word of mouth is so strong." A consultant for Staar in addition to his medical practice, Dougherty now trains surgeons on the procedure and is involved in clinical trials to expand the lens' approved uses to also treat farsightedness. Since becoming involved with Staar, Dougherty now consults for other firms and venture capitalists.

"It's really been synergistic in building my business," said Dougherty, who studied at the Jules Stein Eye Institute at UCLA's Geffen School of Medicine and was one of the first U.S. surgeons to perform laser vision correction on an investigational basis before it was approved by the U.S. Food and Drug Administration in 1995.

"I have a good market advantage because I work with industry," he said. "This is a very high-tech industry, and patients want the latest thing. I don't jump on board every new technology, but I know I've gotten lucky with the ICL."

New Staar Implantable Lens for Nearsightedness Available at Dougherty Laser Vision First Bilateral Implant of FDA-Approved Visian ICL to Be Performed January 13th

Yahoo Finance

Los Angeles, CA, January 12, 2006

Dougherty Laser Vision—one of Southern California's leading centers for vision correction research—is the first surgery center in the Western U.S. to offer the newly FDA-approved Staar Visian ICL (Implantable Collamer Lens) for treating nearsightedness.

The first bilateral (two-eyes) implant of the Visian ICL in the United States following the FDA's December 23rd approval of the lens will be performed on Friday, January 13th at Dougherty Laser Vision's Los Angeles surgery center. Dougherty Laser Vision serves as a principal training center for ophthalmologists seeking to become certified in using the new lens. The first unilateral (single eye) implant of the ICL was performed earlier this week in Wisconsin.

Intended specifically for patients with moderate to severe nearsightedness (myopia that requires -3 to

-20 diopters of correction), the Visian ICL is designed to provide a permanent alternative to glasses/contact lenses, earlier-generation lens implants and LASIK surgery. Procedures such as LASIK, which correct vision by reshaping the cornea, may be considered ill-suited for treating the estimated 34 million Americans with three or more diopters of nearsightedness.

"The new Staar Visian ICL can provide nearsighted patients with many advantages over other available treatment options," said Medical Director

Paul J. Dougherty, M.D. "The medical and aesthetic benefits of this state-of-the-art lens are truly remarkable."

Made of Staar's proprietary, highly biocompatible Collamer material, the Visian ICL can be folded in a manner that allows implantation with an incision up to 50 percent smaller than competing technology.

This surgical benefit may allow for a faster recovery of vision, as well as a reduced risk of inducing astigmatism, which can be a byproduct of earlier generation lens implants for nearsightedness. The Visian lens has what is described as "shape memory," which allows it to be folded into a tiny roll, inserted through an incision just 3 millimeters in length and then unfolded once it is in the eye.

The unique design also allows the lens to be positioned beneath the iris (colored part of the eye), which minimizes risk to the cornea (the clear window in the front of the eye responsible for bending light into focus). The small incision and posterior lens placement combine to provide highly predictable outcomes, while making the lens virtually undetectable to observers. The Visian ICL is designed to remain in the eye permanently, but can be removed or exchanged if a patient's vision changes.

"The ICL's unique foldable design makes it the only minimally invasive lens of its kind approved in the U.S.," added Dr. Dougherty. "The fact that it does not alter the natural shape of the eye means that it has the potential to provide better quality of vision than procedures such as LASIK, especially for patients with higher prescriptions."

The Visian ICL is the result of nearly 15 years of development and international testing. It has been implanted in more than 40,000 eyes worldwide, and is currently approved for use in 41 nations (including the European Union).

While the Food and Drug Administration approved the lens on December 23rd, it will not be available widely in the U.S. until early April.

Dr. Dougherty has implanted the Staar Visian ICL internationally and on an investigational basis in the U.S. for more than six years. He served as a principal investigator for the three-year U.S. clinical trial, and is one of a small handful of surgeons in the U.S. currently trained and certified to implant the lens prior to its commercial release. In addition, Dougherty Laser Vision serves as host to the first post-FDA approval ICL training course for U.S. surgeons. The training course, which will be attended by 40-50 refractive surgeons from across the U.S., will be held on Friday, January 13th at Dougherty Laser Vision's Los Angeles surgery center.

Nearsightedness (myopia) is an error of visual focusing that makes distant objects appear blurred. Like farsightedness (hyperopia) and astigmatism, it is a common refractive error that occurs when the shape of the eye does not bend (i.e. refract) light correctly. Nearsightedness usually develops during childhood, as the eyeball grows too long, and therefore focuses light from distant objects in front of, rather than on, the retina. Nearsightedness affects about one in four people (about 73 million Americans).

Zooming in on Vision Correction
How to Weigh Various Surgery, Spending Options

CBS Marketwatch Online

San Francisco, CA

August 19, 2004

Consumers looking for the right medical and financial fit for vision correction surgery can go cross-eyed considering all the options.

Lasik is by far the most popular procedure that surgically corrects most kinds of nearsightedness, farsightedness and astigmatism, with both traditional and "custom" Lasik accounting for 90 percent of vision-correction surgery.

But it isn't cheap, is rarely covered by insurance and patients with certain visual characteristics aren't candidates for the procedure.

As workers with prescription eyewear take stock of the remaining balances in their pretax flexible-spending accounts, many are considering whether to have vision-correction surgery, what kind is right for them and whether it pays to delay taking action until next year.

Americans pay $3,570 on average to have LASIK surgery on both eyes and they dig up to $800 deeper into their pockets to have the newer wavefront-guided LASIK procedure, said Dave Harmon, president of Market Scope, an ophthalmology industry research firm in St. Louis. Patients are typically in their late 30s and early 40s, he said.

When Lasik first received approval in 1996, "complication rates, though still low, were much higher than they are now," Harmon said, noting that doctors have become better at screening patients.

Those considering pursuing Lasik or other vision-correction surgery are wise not to put it off in hope of seeing major advances just around the corner, he said. "I don't see dramatic improvements on the horizon. I see small, incremental improvements over time."

Weighing cost vs. benefit

Though the upfront fee can be substantial, surgery often drastically cuts spending on glasses and contacts over time, said Dr. Steven E. Wilson, corneal research director and staff refractive surgeon at the Cleveland Clinic's Cole Eye Institute.

"There is a financial savings," Wilson said. "Usually people do this for quality of life [reasons], but as a side benefit you do reduce the cost of taking care of your eyes."

Americans spend about $2 billion a year on refractive surgery, according to Market Scope. They're expected to have 1.3 million procedures this year, up from 1.15 million last year, Harmon said.

As more people consider having laser surgery to shed their glasses and contact lenses, many will find a host of new variations. Here's a look at the latest techniques on the market, their prices and how to tell which one's for you, according to vision-correction experts.

1. Lasik

Lasik surgery, short for laser-assisted in situ keratomileusis, begins by using a microkeratome blade to peel back the outer layers of the eye so the doctor can reshape the cornea underneath with an excimer laser. This flap reattaches to the eye's surface.

The procedure, known as "flap and zap" among ophthalmologists, generally takes three minutes for each eye and requires several hours to recover your vision, said Dr. Paul Dougherty, a clinical instructor at UCLA's Jules Stein Eye Institute. "It's not painful when it's happening, but some people can get some discomfort within the first four to six hours," he said.

2. IntraLase

Refers to Lasik surgery that uses a laser to make the flap that lifts the outer eye layers during the first part of the operation instead of the microkeratome blade used in traditional Lasik. There is some conflicting research on this option.

Some studies suggest patients who opt for IntraLase have fewer complications and less need to have a follow-up enhancement, Harmon said. Still, some patients have a higher incidence of inflammation under the flap after surgery, Dougherty said.

Perhaps the biggest benefit is psychological for patients squeamish about using a blade, Wilson said. "In some cases, that's the major advantage of the procedure—it gets by a block that some patients have about laser vision correction."

Patients may prefer IntraLase, but they'll often pay a premium for it. "The major downside is it's more expensive," Wilson said. "We charge $300 more an eye for it."

3. Wavefront-guided or Custom Lasik

A more precise form of Lasik that involves measuring how the eye bends to 200 points of light as opposed to one point in the middle of the eye in conventional Lasik, said Dr. Robert Maloney, spokesman for the American Academy of Ophthalmology. "The pattern of visual impairment in your eye is as different as your fingerprint," he said. "We can literally customize surgery and that makes it more accurate."

Custom Lasik patients are less likely to need a touch-up and report better night vision than conventional Lasik patients, Maloney said.

Custom treatment isn't yet available for farsighted patients but is expected to be approved by the end of the year, he said. People with thin corneas also may not be candidates.

The extra labor and equipment involved may drive up the price by an additional several hundred dollars per eye. Some doctors assure conventional Lasik patients concerned about having halos that custom treatment is available as a backup, Dougherty said. "I tell my patients we can use it as a safety net if you can only afford conventional."

VISX (EYE: news, chart, profile) is the market leader in wavefront-guided Lasik surgery, accounting for 60 percent of lasers used compared with 20 percent provided by Alcon (ACL: news, chart, profile), Harmon said. The remaining 20 percent of custom lasers are supplied by Nidek, Bausch & Lomb (BOL: news, chart, profile), WaveLight Laser AG and LaserSight, he said.

4. Photorefractive Keratectomy or PRK

This procedure was available prior to Lasik and remains an alternative for many people, especially those with certain eye conditions or thinner corneas, Wilson said. A doctor removes the eye's surface skin with eye drops and performs the corneal reshaping with a laser, though without creating a flap.

The downside is PRK causes more pain and is slower to heal. It typically costs the same as conventional Lasik surgery. Another form of PRK is called Lasek, or laser-assisted subepithelial keratectomy.

5. Conductive Keratoplasty or CK

Those who are over 40 and are farsighted or have presbyopia can have this procedure that uses radio waves to change the shape of the cornea through heat.

Designed to improve reading vision, CK is similar in price to Lasik or PRK, but the effect often disappears over time and some ophthalmologists don't offer it. Wilson and Dougherty said they had reservations about the procedure and don't offer it to patients.

New generation lenses

Patients with visual impairments outside the acceptable range for Lasik surgery or who have early cataracts may be candidates for implantable contacts lenses known as ICLs or intraocular contact lenses called IOLs, Dougherty said. The U.S. Food and Drug Administration is expected to approve the first of these implantable lenses at any time.

One that's already been approved is Crystalens from Eyeonics, the first accommodating replacement lens to provide clear vision at all distances because it's flexible and works with the eye muscles, Dougherty said.

To be sure, the Crystalens procedure is pricey—Dougherty charges $5,000 per eye—and has to be done in a surgery center instead of in the doctor's office.

The Cleveland Clinic's Cole Eye Institute is taking a wait-and-see attitude toward the new generation lenses known as Phakic IOLs, Wilson said.

While recent trials suggest the lenses now have fewer complications than they did earlier, "I think we need much longer follow-up to know how safe this is for someone who's 20 years old," Wilson said. "We plan on approaching this with caution."

Most accommodating and adjustable lenses, which will change shape by shining UV light on the lens, are still five to 10 years from becoming mainstream options, said Maloney of the American Academy of Ophthalmology.

"The problem with any lens or surgery including Lasik is it's not perfectly accurate," Maloney said. "You're never sure you're going to get 20/20. You may still have a little nearsightedness or farsightedness or astigmatism."

Ultimately, patients need to consult with their doctors and take into account their prescriptions, the type of visual problem they have, their age and visual needs to determine which correction makes the most sense to pursue, Dougherty said.

———

Those shopping for a surgeon are wise to choose one who does the pre-operative and post-operative exams as well as performing the surgery, Wilson said.

Patient Testimonials

Over the years, Dr. Dougherty has developed a reputation as "the doctor's doctor" due to the many healthcare professionals who have selected Dougherty Laser Vision for their vision correction needs. Here's what a few of our patients have to say about their experience:

Dear Dr. Dougherty,

I want to thank you for the LASIK treatment you performed on my eyes. I have had absolutely no problems, and my vision is perfect; 20/20 in each eye!

As a practicing optometrist in Ventura for the past 34 years, I recognize that you are one of the foremost eye surgeons in the United States. That is why I recommend you to all of my patients.

Complementing your reputation is your fabulous staff. I was treated like family and every step along the process of my surgery was fully explained. There were no "surprises" at any time. This is of great comfort to patients going through eye surgery—even doctors!

The fact that I experienced no pain, and that my vision went from being "legally blind" before surgery to 20/20 vision on day one post-op, was miraculous!

Thanks again for taking such great care of me.

Robert Pazen, OD

Optometrist

Ventura, California

* * *

Dear Dr. Dougherty,

As an ophthalmic surgeon myself, I was very impressed with your surgical skills and reputation, which I had been aware of for some time. In fact, several years ago I promised myself that if I ever had LASIK performed on my own eyes, you would be my surgeon no matter how far I had to travel. I kept that promise, and the results of the procedure were stunning. The first day after LASIK, I had perfect uncorrected visual acuity. Two weeks later, I was back in Switzerland performing cataract surgery. My vision is perfect.

Peter Trueb, MD

Ophthalmologist

Zurich, Switzerland

* * *

Dear Dr. Dougherty,

I just want to thank you for performing my LASIK. I have had an outstanding result; I was able to go to work the next day, seeing a full load of patients. Two days after the surgery, I was back to performing LASIK on my own patients. It is truly a miracle.

As an ophthalmologist myself, I searched carefully and thoughtfully for the right surgeon to perform the procedure on me. I was extremely impressed with your attention to detail and your outstanding staff. I would highly recommend Dougherty Laser Vision to anyone considering refractive surgery.

Steven O. Rimmer, MD

Ophthalmologist

Redlands, California

* * *

Dear Dr. Dougherty,

I greatly appreciate the gift of vision you have given me. Prior to surgery, my vision was so poor that I couldn't recognize people in the pool until they were virtually bumping heads.

I'd been to other offices in the past and rejected the surgeons due to the lack of informed consent. I felt the discussion of risk you provided was excellent. You made me feel very reassured during surgery. The next morning my vision was 20/20, and I was back in the office seeing patients. The following week my vision improved to 20/15. I can now see waves coming and wind surfing is even more of a rush!

David White, MD
Family Medicine
Ventura, California

* * *

Dear Dr. Dougherty,

I can't thank you enough for my new vision. What a life-changing experience! I keep thinking that it was just too easy. My vision changed dramatically in a matter of hours, and I am now completely free from glasses and contacts for the first time since I can remember.

Thank you. Thank you. Thank you!

Valery Sanchez
Ophthalmic Technician
Santa Barbara, California

* * *

Dear Dr. Dougherty,

I decided to have LASIK surgery after having worn glasses since the age of six. My vision was roughly 20/400 when I contacted your office for an evaluation. You had come highly recommended by several of my colleagues.

Your exam was thorough and the time you spent explaining the procedure and answering my questions was more than adequate. The follow-up care was excellent, and my outcome was perfect.

I strong recommend Dougherty Laser Vision to anyone considering LASIK.

Ray Greek, MD
Anesthesiologist
Goleta, California

* * *

Dear Dr. Dougherty,

I want to thank you for giving me the gift of 20/20 vision, which I have not experienced since grade school. The surgery was so quick and painless. It's hard to believe that I could walk into the office with 20/500 vision, and walk out seeing 20/20.

I also want to thank your great staff for making me feel very comfortable and confident in your services. Eye surgery can be a very scary thing, but I would certainly recommend Dougherty Laser Vision.

Anita Shaffer
Office Manager
Oxnard, California

* * *

Dear Dr. Dougherty,

As an artist, I need to plan each new painting with a foreground, middle ground and background. Thank you for giving me the ability to clearly see all of them with the surgery you performed on my eyes. The result was all that you promised.

Sue Govelon
Artist
Thousand Oaks, California

* * *

Dr. Dougherty,

As an eye care professional, I have had an abundance of vision correction options available to me. I was legally blind without correction, and have depended on glasses and contact lenses for the past seventeen years in order to function.

My glasses simply got in the way while examining my patients, exercising, and going about my daily activities. I have always advised my patients who sleep in their contacts, or have presented with contact lens related problems like infections, ulcers, or neo-vascularization to go have a consultation with you for LASIK since this is a safer alternative.

When the time came for me to choose a surgeon, there was no question as to whom I trusted with my eyes. This eye doctor was very anxious prior to surgery. You and your wonderful staff quickly put me at ease. I was a perfect 20/20 and back to work in less than 24 hours.

Thank you for taking such excellent care of me!

Anne E. Savko, O.D.

Optometrist

Thousand Oaks, California

Glossary

Aberration: Distortions in the eye that bend light rays entering the eye in unpredictable ways so that all the rays do not come to a single point focus on the retina. Aberrations are divided into two main categories: higher-order and lower-order.

Ablation: Surgical removal of tissue, typically using a cool laser beam.

Accommodation: Ability of the eye to change its focus between distant objects and near objects; zooming power of the eye.

Acuity: Sharpness, acuteness, or keenness of vision.

Acute: Of short duration; occurring suddenly.

Age-Related Macular Degeneration (ARMD): Common age-related disease of the retina that results in disruption of the photoreceptors and loss of vision. Two types exist: dry ARMD that manifests as drusen (age spots) and loss of pigment cells of the retina. Wet ARMD is the more serious form that manifests as development of blood vessels and loss of vision.

Amblyopia (lazy eye): Dullness or reduction of sight for no apparent organic reason, therefore not correctable with glasses or surgery. Sometimes called a lazy eye, where one eye becomes dependent on the other eye to focus; usually developed in early childhood. Amblyopia is often associated with strabismus (crossed eyes).

Anisometropia: When both eyes have unequal refractive power.

Anterior chamber: Space between the cornea and the lens, which contains aqueous humor.

Aphakia: Absence of the lens of the eye.

Astigmatism: A visual abnormality in which the optical surface of the eye (the cornea) is shaped like a football (oval) rather than a basketball (round), resulting in images from an object not meeting in a single focal point.

Astigmatism blurs vision for both distance and near objects. Astigmatism can occur alone, but is most often combined with myopia or hyperopia.

Axis: The direction of astigmatism.

Best corrected visual acuity (BCVA): Best possible vision a person can achieve with corrective lenses, measured on an eye chart.

Bifocals: Lenses containing two focal lengths, usually arranged with the focus for distance above and near focus below.

Binocular vision: Simultaneous use of the two eyes. Normal binocular vision yields a stereoscopic image and parallax-induced depth perception.

Capsular bag: The membrane surrounding the crystalline lens, which is left in place at the time of cataract surgery to hold the intraocular lens (IOL). The capsular bag frequently becomes cloudy soon after cataract surgery—see PCO.

Cataract: Gradual clouding of the crystalline lens resulting in reduced vision, correctable by cataract surgery. Cataracts are usually age-related, but can be caused at an earlier age by trauma, steroid use, high nearsightedness, or diabetes.

Cataract surgery: Removal of a cataract with ultrasound (phacoemulsification), replacing it with an intraocular lens implant.

Chronic: Of long duration; going on for some time.

Ciliary muscle (ciliary body): Muscle attached to the crystalline lens responsible for focus (accommodation).

Clear Lens Extraction (CLE): Procedure in which the eye's natural clear crystalline lens is removed and replaced with an intraocular lens implant using the same technique as cataract surgery. CLE is also known as Refractive Lens Exchange/Lensectomy (RLE).

CME: Cystoid macular edema. Swelling of the central portion of the retina that can blur vision after IOL implantation.

Conjunctiva: The clear mucous membrane lining the sclera (white of the eye) and the inner surface of the eyelids that is responsible for keeping the eye moist.

Conjunctivitis: Inflammation or irritation of the conjunctiva. Symptoms can be present in just one eye, or it can affect both eyes and include redness of the eyes or the edges of the eyelids, swelling of the eyelids, or itching.

Contact lens: Small, thin, removable plastic lens worn directly on the front of the eyeballs, usually used instead of ordinary eyeglasses for correction of vision.

Contrast sensitivity: A measure of visual sharpness, specifically the ability to distinguish visual details under varying contrast conditions.

Cornea: The clear window in front of the eye that covers the iris and pupil. The cornea is the first part of the eye that bends (or refracts) incoming light and provides most of the focusing power of the eye.

Corneal curvature: Shape of the front of the eye.

Corneal mapping/corneal topography: An instrument used to see the curvature of the cornea. Corneal topography is used not only for screening all patients before refractive surgery like LASIK but also for fitting contacts.

Corneal transplant (penetrating keratoplasty): Surgical operation of grafting a replacement cornea onto an eye.

Custom treatment: LASIK or PRK treatment of eyes that incorporates both the prescription and the specific aberrations of the eye.

Crystalens: A type of accommodating (flexing) intraocular lens implant.

Crystalline lens: Double convex, transparent part of the eye, located behind the iris and in front of the vitreous body. Serves in conjunction with the cornea to bend (refract) incoming rays of light onto the retina.

Cylinder: Refers to the degree of astigmatism present in the eye.

Depth perception: Ability of the vision system to perceive the relative positions of objects in the visual field.

Detached retina: See retinal detachment.

Diabetes mellitus: Chronic metabolic disorder characterized by a lack of insulin secretion and/or increased cellular resistance to insulin, resulting in elevated blood levels of simple sugars (glucose) and including complications involving damage to the eyes, kidneys, nervous system, and vascular system.

Diabetes type I (IDDM): Insulin dependent, resulting from destruction of the insulin producing pancreatic islet cells.

Diabetes type II (NIDDM): Non-insulin dependent, resulting from tissue resistance to insulin.

Diabetic retinopathy: Deterioration of retinal blood vessels in diabetic patients, possibly leading to vision loss.

Dilation: Enlargement of the pupil (the opening in the middle of the iris).

Diopter: Unit of measure of the refractive power of an optical lens or the eye. A negative diopter value (such as -3D) signifies an eye with myopia and positive diopter value (such as +3D) signifies an eye with hyperopia.

Dry eye: A common condition that occurs when the eyes do not produce enough tears or the correct type of tears to keep the eye moist and comfortable.

Ectasia: Progressive steepening and thinning of the cornea that rarely occurs after LASIK that can require Intacs, a hard contact lens or cornea transplant to regain clear vision.

Emmetropia: An eye that has no refractive error and therefore does not need glasses or contact lenses to see clearly.

Endothelium: The layer of cells that covers the inner surface of the cornea that helps maintain the clarity of the cornea by pumping excess water out of the cornea.

Enhancement: An additional surgical procedure used to refine the results of the original refractive surgery.

Epithelium: The layer of cells that covers the outer surface of the eye.

Excimer laser: Laser used in LASIK and PRK surgery that operates in the ultraviolet wavelength, producing a cool beam to remove tissue without the production of heat.

Eye chart: Technically called a Snellen chart, a printed visual acuity chart consisting of Snellen optotypes, which are specifically formed letters of the alphabet arranged in rows of decreasing letter size.

Eyelid: Either of two movable, protective folds of flesh that cover and uncover the front of the eyeball.

Farsighted: Common term for hyperopia. Farsighted patients first lose their near vision, but will also eventually lose their far vision as they age.

FDA: Abbreviation for the Food and Drug Administration. It is the United States governmental agency responsible for the evaluation and approval of drugs and medical devices.

Femtosecond laser: A laser used to create a flap in LASIK without the need for a metal blade, typically resulting in a safer and more precise flap than older metal blade technology. Two types of femtosecond lasers are currently available in the United States: the older IntraLase and the newer Ziemer LDV laser (that allows for the first true all-laser LASIK).

Flap: A round-hinged portion of the top three layers of the cornea (epithelium, Bowman's membrane, and some stroma) that is created by a femtosecond laser or mechanical keratome during the LASIK procedure. The flap is lifted up and the excimer laser corrects for the prescription of the eye by reshaping the corneal stroma beneath the flap.

Giant papillary conjunctivitis (GPC): Type of conjunctivitis wherein bumps or ridges form on the inside of eyelids, which make wearing contact lenses uncomfortable; in fact, this condition is often caused by over-wearing of certain contact lenses.

Glare: Scatter from bright light that decreases vision.

Glaucoma: Painless disease of the eye characterized by increased pressure within the eye. If the high pressure is left untreated it leads to a gradual impairment of sight, often resulting in blindness.

Halos: Rings around lights due to optical imperfections in the eye.

Herpes: A recurrent viral infection caused by the herpes simplex virus. Ocular herpes represents the most common infectious cause of corneal blindness in the United States.

Haptics: The arms of an intraocular lens that holds it in place in the capsular bag of the eye.

Haze: Clouding of the cornea that can occasionally occur after PRK that may or may not blur vision.

Hyperopia: Also called farsightedness, hyperopia is the inability to see near objects as clearly as distant objects, and the need for accommodation to see distant objects clearly.

ICL (also known as the Visian ICL): Implantable collamer lens or implantable contact lens. A lens made of biocompatible collamer material that is placed between the normal lens of the eye and back of the cornea for patients with low to high nearsightedness.

Image: Light reflected into the eye, off of objects in front of the eye. This light contains all the information about the objects (such as color, shadow, motion, and detail) that are translated to the brain and allow you to "see" (know about the objects).

Implantable collamer lens: See implantable contact lens or ICL.

Implantable contact lens: See ICL.

Inflammation: Body's reaction to trauma, infection, or a foreign substance, often associated with pain, heat, redness, swelling, and/or loss of function.

Informed consent form: Document disclosing the risks, benefits, and alternatives to a procedure.

Intacs: Surgically implanted plastic half rings that change the shape of the cornea that are used to treat keratoconus and ectasia.

Intraocular lens implant (IOL): Permanent, artificial lens surgically inserted inside the eye to replace the crystalline lens following cataract surgery or clear lens extraction.

Intraocular pressure (IOP): Fluid pressure within the eye created by the continual production and drainage of aqueous fluid in the anterior chamber. Normal IOP is 8-22.

Iridotomy: Surgical opening performed at the time of ICL surgery in the iris to allow fluid to flow normally and prevent angle-closure glaucoma.

Iris: Colored part of the eye. Elastic, pigmented, muscular tissue in front of the crystalline lens that regulates the amount of light that enters the eye by adjusting the size of the pupil in the center.

Irregular astigmatism: An irregular curvature of the cornea.

Keratectomy: Surgical removal of corneal tissue.

Keratotomy: Surgical incision (cut) of the cornea.

Keratoconus: Rare, serious, degenerative corneal disease, which creates a progressive steepening and thinning of the cornea so that the cornea assumes the shape of a cone and blurs vision.

Keratomileusis: Carving of the cornea to reshape it.

Keratoplasty: Surgical reshaping of the cornea.

LASEK: Laser Epithelial Keratomileusis—a type of PRK where alcohol is used to remove the epithelium rather than a spatula. Only used when surface laser treatment is performed over a previous LASIK flap in order to preserve the integrity of the underlying flap.

Laser: Device that generates an intense and highly concentrated beam of light. Acronym for: Light Amplification by Simulated Emission of Radiation. (Also see: YAG laser, femtosecond laser, and excimer laser.)

LASIK: The most common refractive surgery procedure performed in the world. An acronym for Laser-Assisted In Situ Keratomileusis, a refractive surgery in which Excimer laser ablation is performed under a flap on the cornea to correct refractive errors.

Lazy eye: See amblyopia.

Legally blind: 20/200 vision or worse is the qualification of legal blindness in the United States.

Lens: Same as the crystalline lens. Double convex, clear part of the eye, behind the iris and in front of the vitreous humor that serves to refract the various rays of light so as to form an image on the retina.

Lensectomy: Removal of the natural lens of the eye with ultrasound.

LRI: Limbal relaxing incisions—small incisions placed in the far periphery of the cornea, typically at the time of IOL or ICL surgery, to correct astigmatism by relaxing the steep axis of the cornea.

Limbus: Thin area that connects the cornea and the sclera.

Macula: Yellow spot on the retina, where the photoreceptors are most dense and responsible for the central vision. Has the greatest concentration of cones; responsible for visual acuity and the ability to see in color.

Macular edema: See CME.

Macular degeneration: Disease of the macula, which results in the loss of central vision. Can be related to aging (ARMD: age-related macular degeneration) or due to high myopia.

Microkeratome: Mechanical surgical device that is affixed to the eye by use of a vacuum ring. When secured, a laser or very sharp blade cuts a layer of the cornea at a predetermined depth.

Monovision: Purposeful adjustment of one eye for near vision and the other eye for distance vision. Also known as blended vision.

Myopia: Also called nearsightedness or shortsightedness, the inability to see distant objects as clearly as near objects.

Nanoflex: A type of accommodating (flexing) intraocular lens implant.

Nearsighted: Common term for myopia.

Normal vision: Also known as emmetropia. Occurs when light is focused directly on the retina rather than in front or behind it so that the eye can see without glasses or contacts.

OD: The right eye—abbreviation for "oculus dextrum."

OS: The left eye—abbreviation for "oculus sinister."

OU: Both eyes.

Off-label: Use of a drug or device in a way that is not specifically approved or disapproved by the FDA. Off-label uses are very common throughout the practice of medicine.

Ophthalmologist (MD): An ophthalmologist is a medical doctor (MD) who is qualified and especially trained to diagnose and treat all eye and visual system problems, both medically and surgically, as well as diagnose general diseases of the body.

Optician: Expert who designs, verifies, and dispenses lenses, frames, and other fabricated optical devices upon the prescription of an ophthalmologist or an optometrist.

Optometrist (OD): Eye care professional, graduate of optometry school, provides non-surgical vision care. Specifically educated and trained to examine the eyes, and determine visual acuity as well as other vision problems and ocular abnormalities. An optometrist prescribes glasses and contact lenses to improve visual acuity and performs care before and after eye surgery.

Overcorrection: Occurrence in refractive surgery where the achieved amount of correction is more than desired; occurs in LASIK or PRK, typically due to a patient's over-response to the laser ablation.

Pellucid marginal degeneration: A form of keratoconus that involves a progressive thinning of the lower part of the cornea resulting in a "lobster claw" pattern on topography.

Phakic Intraocular Lens (Phakic IOL): A lens placed inside the eye without removing the natural lens, and performs much like an internal contact lens. See ICL and Verisys.

Phoropter: A common device with multiple lenses, found in most eye doctors' offices and used to measure refractive errors. A phoropter calculates the prescription required for corrective lenses.

Photophobia: Sensitivity to light.

Photorefractive Keratectomy (PRK): Also known as flapless LASIK, PRK is a type of refractive surgery in which the corneal epithelial cells (surface cells) are gently removed and the excimer laser reshapes the corneal surface.

Posterior Capsular Opacity (PCO): Clouding of the back portion of the capsular bag that occurs after cataract surgery or refractive lens exchange that blurs vision. PCO is extremely common after IOL surgery and is caused by growth of microscopic cells left in the capsular bag after the crystalline lens has been removed. PCO is treated by using a YAG laser to clean the cloudy capsule behind the IOL.

Presbyopia: The age-related loss of zooming power of the eye resulting in the inability to maintain a clear image (focus) as objects are moved closer. Presbyopia is due to reduced elasticity of the lens with increasing age.

Prescription: Amount of vision correction necessary, written in a form that can be used to create eyeglasses or to program the excimer laser prior to LASIK surgery.

PRK: Acronym for Photo-Refractive Keratectomy, which is a procedure involving the removal of the surface layer of the cornea (epithelium) by gentle brushing and use of an excimer laser to reshape the stroma.

Pupil: Black, circular opening in the center of the iris through which light passes into the crystalline lens. It changes size in response to how much light is being received by the eye—larger in dim lighting conditions and smaller in brighter lighting conditions.

Radial Keratotomy (RK): Outdated procedure once used to correct mild to moderate nearsightedness, by making a series of spoke-like incisions around the periphery of the cornea to flatten it.

Refract: To bend light, as in "the crystalline lens refracts the light as it passes through," or to measure the degree the eye or a lens bends light, as in "the doctor refracts a patient's eyes."

Refraction: Test to determine the refractive power of the eye; also, the bending of light as it passes from one medium into another.

Refractive errors: The degree of visual distortion or limitation caused by inadequate bending of light rays; includes hyperopia, myopia, and astigmatism.

Refractive Lens Exchange (RLE): Removing the natural lens and replacing it with an IOL to treat nearsightedness, farsightedness, and/or astigmatism.

Refractive power: Ability of an object, such as the eye, to bend light as light passes through it.

Refractive surgery: Type of surgery (such as LASIK) that changes the ability of the eye to bend light in order to minimize the need for glasses or contacts.

Regression: Complication of refractive surgery, most commonly LASIK or PRK, where the eye heals back towards its original refractive error.

Restor: A type of multi-focal IOL that splits light into distance and near components to decrease the need for both distance and near glasses.

Retina: Layer of fine sensory tissue that lines the inside wall of the eye, composed of light sensitive cells known as rods and cones. Acts like the film in a camera to capture images; transforms the images into electrical signals, and sends the signals to the brain by way of the optic nerve.

Retinal detachment: Condition wherein the retina breaks away from the inside of the eye, causing it to lose nourishment and resulting in loss of vision unless successfully surgically repaired.

RK: Outdated procedure once used to correct mild to moderate nearsightedness, by making a series of spoke-like incisions around the periphery of the cornea to flatten it.

Sclera: While part of the eye. Tough covering that (with the cornea) forms the external, protective coat of the eye.

Softec HD: A type of accommodating (flexing) intraocular lens implant that seems to work best for farsighted patients.

Sphere: Focusing power of a corrective lens.

Strabismus: Condition occurs when the muscles of the eye do not align properly and binocular vision is not present.

Stroma: Middle, thickest layer of tissue in the cornea.

Tecnis: A type of multi-focal IOL that splits light into distance and near components to decrease the need for both distance and near glasses.

Topography: See corneal mapping.

Topo-guided: See topography-guided LASIK.

Topography-guided LASIK: LASIK that measures the prescription of the eye and thousands of points on the corneal surface to treat refractive power and unique surface imperfections of the eye.

Twenty-twenty, 20/20 vision: Also known as perfect vision. To have 20/20 vision means that when you stand 20 feet away from the eye chart, you can see what someone who has perfect vision can see from that distance.

UCVA: Uncorrected visual acuity. Measurement of what an eye can see without glasses or contacts.

Ultrasound waves: Sound waves above 20,000 vibrations per second, above the range audible to the human ear; used in medical diagnosis and surgery.

Ultrasonography (UBM): Recordings of the echoes of ultrasound waves sent into the eye and reflected from the structures inside the eye or orbit. Ultrasonography is used by refractive surgeons primarily to measure the length of the eye for IOL calculations, and to measure the width of the inside of the eye to properly size ICLs.

Ultraviolet radiation: Radiant energy with a wavelength just below that of the visible light. UV-c is the shortest wavelength at 200-280 nm, and is absorbed by the atmosphere before reaching the surface. UV-b, at 280-315 nm, is the *burning rays* of the sun and damages most living tissue. UV-a, at 315-400 nm, is the *tanning rays* of the sun and is somewhat damaging to certain tissues. UV radiation has been described as a contributing factor to some eye disease processes, which result in ARMD (age-related macular degeneration) and cataracts and causes exposure keratitis.

Undercorrection: Occurrence in refractive surgery where the achieved amount of correction is less than desired; occurs in LASIK, typically due to a patient's cornea under-responding to the laser treatment.

Verisys: An outdated type of implantable contact lens, which clips to the iris of the eye.

Vision: The ability of the brain to see and interpret what is in front of the eyes.

Visual acuity: Clearness of vision; the ability to distinguish details and shapes, which depends upon the sharpness of the retinal image.

Vitreous humor, fluid, or body: Jelly-like, colorless, transparent substance occupying the greater part of the cavity of the eye, and all the space between the crystalline lens and the retina.

Wavefront: Wavefront technology produces a detailed map of the subtle imperfections of the eye. The information is transferred to the laser via computer software to perform a custom- or wavefront-guided ablation.

YAG laser: Properly called a Nd:YAG (neodymium-yttrium-aluminum-garnet) laser. This laser is used to clear a posterior capsular opacity (PCO) that commonly occurs after IOL implantation in a procedure called a YAG capsulotomy, which takes seconds and is performed in the office.

Index

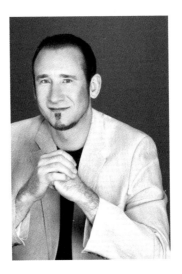

Dr. Paul Dougherty is one of our country's leading pioneers in advanced vision correction surgery. He has helped to develop many lens and laser-based vision correction technologies that have revolutionized his field, often travelling the globe training refractive surgeons in those techniques. His Southern California-based Dougherty Laser Vision is considered a major center for clinical research involving the latest innovations in refractive surgery. Dr. Dougherty devotes a great deal of time to volunteer work, improving the vision of countless impoverished and deserving people across the United States and around the world.